TSUNAMI EFFECT

Timothy L Trujillo

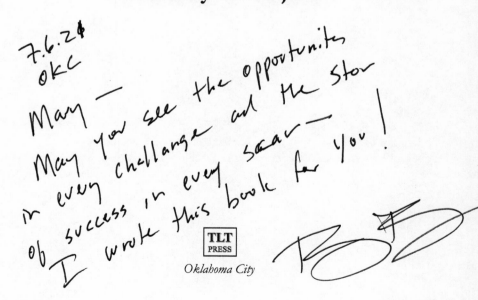

7.6.2$
OKC

May —

May you see the opportunities
in every challange and the Star
of success in every soar —
I wrote this book for you!

TLT PRESS

Oklahoma City

TLT PRESS

An imprint of
TLT PRODUCTIONS LLC
4301 N. Classen Blvd. Ste B
Oklahoma City, Oklahoma 73118
timothytrujillo.com/TLT
310-392-9663

ISBN: 978-0-9907334-0-9

He who saves a life
is as if he has saved the entire world

Babylonian Talmud, Sanhedrin, 37a

For the traveler,
the healer,
and the one in need

Prologue

Each of us is likely to experience a personal catastrophe. An accident, disaster, illness, or death will directly or indirectly impact us at some time. Our response to this event will determine the manner of our short-term recovery and long-term life path. As in that scene in the movie *JAWS*, it is the telling of the stories of our scars that brings meaning to our lives. The first cracks on the egg destroy what was, but they are a harbinger of something new that is emerging.

This is a story about my experience. In 1993 a back injury brought episodes of intense pain and an end to my job, my nearly twenty year career as a performer, and all aspirations of achieving my long sought goals. Following my doctor's advice, I set out to "find something else to do with my life." This led me on a remarkable odyssey of challenge and adventure. Along the way, I learned that it was my own suffering and loss that enabled me to help others in a way that has truly made a difference. My personal disaster, rather than derailing my dreams and goals, set a path of destiny that has changed my world.

I wrote this story to share the unfathomable capacity for healing that I have witnessed. My hope is that a need will be answered in the reading of this tale, just as mine have been through its unfolding. It is the story of the Asian Tsunami of 2004 and its effect on those who endured it and responded to its impact. Throughout this tale is the reflection of how virtually every event in my own life prepared me for these moments of action. Come along with me on this journey now.

1

December 26

December 26 is commonly known as Boxing Day throughout much of the English-speaking world. This, I was told, is due to a long-held custom of packing the remnants of the Christmas feast and cast-off treasures into boxes that were given to the servants and the poor. Since the servants were engaged on Christmas day, on Boxing Day they were given the day to celebrate with family.

I did not learn of this custom until my mid-twenties, but always seeking another holiday to celebrate, I have tried to keep this tradition in some manner, if only by taking the day off. I have frequently followed late holiday reveling on Christmas night with a sleep-in, lounge-around, video-viewing Boxing Day.

On December 26, 2004, I lazily rose from bed and crept to the coffee maker. My wife Lenise and I were house and cat-sitting at our friends John and Sarah Cooke's place in Topanga Canyon. The night before, we had enjoyed our "Island of Lost Toys Christmas Party" at friends Anne Marie and Bernie Wire's. A gathering for those of us living in Los Angeles whose families were in distant cities, it had been our traditional celebration for almost fifteen years.

It was raining when we left their Marina Del Rey neighborhood to make the twenty minute drive. By the time we reached the Topanga Canyon Blvd. turnoff from Pacific Coast Highway, the gentle rain had become a downpour. The winding, climbing, narrow road can be a challenge to navigate at night during the best conditions. However, with some passages so narrow there was only the guardrail between the road and the deep slope to the wrecked-vehicle littered bottom of the canyon, the reduced visibility made the drive a white-knuckled, breathless, feat of endurance. The entire ordeal was worsened by the locals on their familiar roadway, seeming to maneuver effortlessly through all conditions, ultimately gathering as an impatient parade behind us.

Our safe arrival within the secluded compound and dry house was a warm and comforting relief. After tending to the needs of the herd of eight cats, we settled calmly into our rain-serenaded sleep.

The rain continued throughout the night and as I came to my wakeful senses, I noticed that the Topanga Creek flowing directly beside the property had grown from its usual one-foot depth and ten-foot width into a raging torrent. It filled the ravine to a depth of twenty or so feet and expanded to a width of forty to fifty feet. Its normally gentle flow was now a racing, crashing force, and it seemed as though, if it continued to increase, it would eventually take away part of the house itself.

Just then, a knock came at the door. It was a rescue worker searching for a homeless man who had been living beneath the bridge nearby. He had gone missing during the night. A brief examination in the lightly falling rain revealed his sleeping bag tangled in tree branches in the center of the roaring stream. We found no other signs of the man, but the searcher left with diminished hope.

The worst of the storm seemed to be passed, but I wanted to know the forecast in case we would need to evacuate, cats and all. I went to the computer to get weather information and while reading a news site, saw that a massive earthquake had occurred in the Indian Ocean, just off the coast of Sumatra. The next headline predicted an earthquake-induced tsunami. The next headline began to report the tsunami's effect.

A sudden slip in the fault line between the India and Burma Plates had caused 1200 kilometers of ocean floor to drop twenty meters. The shock, with the force of a 22 megaton explosion, jolted the globe and caused the day to be almost three seconds shorter. The massive "kerplunk" as the ocean floor dropped displaced billions of gallons of water and created a ripple from bottom to surface, radiating out at 500 miles per hour.

Soon, television reports announced that a tsunami had struck the coast of Sumatra, then Indonesia, Thailand, Sri Lanka, India, and the eastern tip of Africa. Accounts were foggy, yet dire. Within a few hours, the first images arrived, images of devastation only previously seen in Hiroshima, Nagasaki, and Dresden. An expansive, denuded, yet color-speckled landscape stretched in every direction; no recognizable structures remained, only scattered debris. What first appeared was a silent spectacle of destruction, but soon that was followed by reports of one thousand, ten thousand, one hundred thousand, two hundred thousand dead. The world stopped and wept for the lost.

Within hours the response began. Military forces and volunteers from around the world intervened to prevent an even greater looming threat, a disease outbreak. The precision of cooperation and shared effort between agencies and governments was unprecedented. Then came reports of the flood of donated money and relief supplies. Partly due to the round-the-clock visual news coverage, the very spirit of the season, as well as the overwhelming enormity of the disaster, people opened their accounts and gave graciously to reduce the suffering. So great was the response that Doctors Without Borders, a highly-regarded disaster response agency, began to decline and redirect donations. One seismic event on the ocean floor triggered a tsunami of destruction and an avalanche of compassion.

On December 26, as mentioned, we were house-sitting in Topanga canyon. Lenise and I were preparing for a trip to Guatemala to deliver a series of self-care workshops for adults and children affected by HIV/AIDS through our organization First Medicines. Our lives were in a limbo world of house-sits and fundraising projects. On December 28 a donation arrived at the office that completed our budget for the Guatemala trip. In the spirit of Boxing Day, we were gathering donated goodies for a rummage sale as part of our Guatemala fundraising efforts. Since we had met our fundraising goals, we decided to divert half of the proceeds of the sale to some type of tsunami relief. As we began our planning, I also grew eager to find a good program for which our humble gift of a few hundred dollars would make a significant difference, just as it would for our own project.

I began to discuss this notion with others. Some days later, while sharing my idea with a colleague, Ryan Gierach, he mentioned that a friend of his had set up a fund for a family in a tsunami-affected village in India. A few days after that my phone rang; it was Ryan's friend Jim Rudolph.

Jim began to describe the plight of the people in this far away place. He told me of a family he had been adopted into thirty years earlier. He related how he had seen the family grow and change over time, and how he had sponsored educational needs for members of the family. The son in the family, Dhamodharan, had just completed his Masters Degree in Computer Arts with his support. He then told me that on December 26 the family had been devastated by the tsunami. Though all family members escaped alive and with little harm, all of their possessions had been claimed by the sea. He was gathering funds to help them restore their lives and lend support to others in the village affected by the disaster.

Jim also told me that in addition to many homes being destroyed and many lives lost in this village, they were a village of fishermen whose boats had been destroyed. They were not just without homes and belongings, their very method of making money to restore these needs had also been taken from them. Recovery would be a long and deeply challenged process while lacking their very means of daily survival, their catch from the sea.

I had already been emotionally moved by the level of trauma I observed in the survivors interviewed on television. My heart was drawn to the need for trauma recovery, one of my therapeutic specialties. I had ruminated on some way to help, perhaps by offering our funds to a trauma intervention team or presenting workshops for relief workers who also seemed to exhibit signs of overwhelm and despair. As I spoke with Jim, an idea came to mind.

I told Jim of Dr. Mikao Usui and the hands-on energy healing system known as Reiki. According to legend, when Dr. Usui first developed his simple system of Reiki in the early 1900s, he taught it to the beggars of Tokyo. As an alternative to begging, he told them to give treatments to others and accept their gifts of food and money in exchange. I asked Jim if he thought that giving these same tools to some of the members of the village may also give them a tradable skill. It would also provide enduring therapeutic mechanisms within the community to reduce suffering, which is the primary mission of First Medicines. Jim was open to this idea. He certainly felt that it merited further consideration. We scheduled a meeting to talk.

2

Turning on a Dime

We had planned to hold our rummage sale on January 8 in order to receive Boxing Day donations and have plenty of time to organize them. Rain came on the 8th instead and we were happy to postpone the sale to the weekend of the 15th. We were scheduled to depart for Guatemala on the 24th, so there was no concern regarding the delay. It was on the 8th that I first spoke with Jim Rudolph. Lenise had stepped out of the office for lunch with a client. When she returned, I informed her of the call. It seemed a radical notion to shift the trip from Guatemala to India. We had not yet purchased our airplane tickets, so we would not lose money, but shifting the trip would be no small action.

Years in development, the trip was to be a pilot project to demonstrate the effectiveness of mind-body self-care therapies for individuals affected by HIV/AIDS. I had initiated the work in Hollywood in 1996 through a series of self-hypnosis workshops at AIDS Project Los Angeles. I developed a practical, evidence-based protocol to help participants manage stress, pain, sleep, treatment side effects, and emotional trauma related to diagnosis and life with HIV infection. The success of the Hypnosis AIDS Project drove me to seek a way to deliver these methods beyond the Los Angeles community. In the absence of current anti-retroviral therapies in the developing world, I felt they could make a difference for those suffering.

In July of 2002, I was given the opportunity to share my work at the United Nations. Wilda Spalding, founder of the International Human

Rights Consortium (IHRC), invited me to speak at a "Healthcare in Crisis" roundtable discussion during a U.N. Human Rights Commission meeting in Geneva, Switzerland. After my presentation, I was told by an official from UNAIDS that my program seemed sound and she understood its value. However, it was not enough to simply say that I could make a difference; I needed to conduct a pilot project and report how I had succeeded.

I returned to Geneva with Lenise the following summer. We attended the U.N. Working Group on Indigenous Populations to conduct needs assessment interviews with indigenous leaders from around the world. Through these interviews, I was coached to adapt the hypnosis-centric, AIDS-specific model of our Hypnosis Health Service into a universal program. We would need to be accessible to all persons, with the goal of supporting good health in the face of any challenge.

In the summer of 2004, I traveled to Guatemala on the invitation of Lorenzo and Emilia Gottschammer who operate a macadamia farm and re-forestation project near Antigua. I had met them in Geneva in 2002 while they were being honored by IHRC for delivering over 100,000 macadamia trees to indigenous farmers. I was accompanied by Jeff Neff of Mesoamerican Health Assistance Project of California (MAHAPCA), based in Los Angeles. During the ten day trip, we established a working relationship with a hospital for children with AIDS, an AIDS service organization in the Northwestern frontier, and community leaders in Antigua who would sponsor trainings for the general public. We also enjoyed eating a lot of macadamia nuts and pancakes with fresh blueberry jam. We established a plan to return in the winter to conduct programs.

It was Jeff Neff who first introduced me to the idea of "backyard medicine". He said it was a Mayan philosophy to look for those things that are near and accessible, "in our own backyard", and use them to treat our needs. While in Guatemala, I observed the Mayan sustainable agriculture technique of growing beans up the cornstalk as support while returning nutrients to the soil, along with squash beside to distract the bugs by feeding them the leaves. I found it to be brilliant, especially while growing a whole meal in a single spot. It was this wisdom of the "First Peoples", along with the "Backyard Medicine" that gave birth to First Medicines, and its mission to reduce suffering and enhance health through the cultivation of internal resources applied in a sustainable manner.

When the option arose to postpone the Guatemala trip and travel to India to help tsunami victims, Lenise and I talked at length about the impulsive decision of turning from a long-developed plan to a sudden redirection of both location and mission scope. We were committed to keeping our promise to the people of Guatemala. We both knew the importance of the opportunity and the hazards of traveling into a disaster zone. We also knew that the travel expenses would be higher and probably only allow one of us to take the journey.

Lenise is a remarkable project coordinator; a friend-maker and troubleshooter of the highest order, helping every endeavor go more smoothly. She is also a gifted artist and master garden designer, specializing in planting habitats for birds and butterflies, dressed in the colors of culinary and medicinal herbs. In addition to spending time with Mayan villagers in the Guatemalan highlands, we had also set up a trip to a medicinal herb farm in Honduras. It was the surrender of a grand dream, but Lenise and I both decided we should follow the path of circumstance and take the work to India, even if it meant that I would go alone. It would be important for Lenise to coordinate project details from the U.S. We would postpone our mission together to Guatemala until a later time.

I met with Jim three days later. We spoke more in-depth about the conditions and needs within the village. I painted a detailed picture of the therapies and training I could provide, something he was very familiar with, being a touch therapist himself. He also knew one of my colleagues and program members, Dean Williams, himself a hypnotherapist and my Reiki Master Instructor. In our lengthy, friendly meeting, Jim concluded that this might, indeed, be a meaningful outreach project for his "family" in India. Particularly since it was an education-based outreach, if accepted by the other villagers, it could be a splendid long-term gift to the community. It would also benefit him for us to help Dhamodharan with needs-assessments for the funds that were being sent.

Over the next ten days, I contacted our friends in Guatemala to apologetically postpone our trip, conducted the fundraiser sale with help from several of our project volunteers, secured funds from our sponsors, acquired remedies to help combat the plague of hazards I was warned to expect, and acquired a visa to travel to India. I was admittedly anxious about traveling into the tsunami zone, not knowing what risks I could encounter. The visa process involved attending a day-long session about one hour's drive south of our West Hollywood office. Paperwork was completed in the morning and a long break was given to process and prepare it for distribution in the late afternoon. I decided to see a movie at a nearby theater. Watching the film Ladder 49, I trembled as firefighter Joaquin Phoenix desperately struggled, trapped in a burning building. I could not escape the feeling that it could be a bad omen for my excursion. I was happy that it was only a story, but I had difficulty shaking my own sense of impending risk.

During this ten day period, I also received a call from Mitta Wise, our volunteer Member Services Director. She expressed her desire to accompany me on the trip and travel at her own expense. She is a skilled hypnotherapy and bodywork practitioner as well as a registered nurse. Since it seemed that having a second therapist on the trip with her skills and the ability to cross gender barriers would be highly beneficial, we welcomed her to the team.

I completed my appointments, cleared my calendar for three weeks, and initiated dialogue via email with Dhamodharan. I also conducted a full-day workshop at our Center in West Hollywood. I did this because I had initiated a policy to provide care to the local community before traveling to offer services far away. I maintained that it was not necessary for me to travel great distances to help, as I could crawl to the need from the spot on which I stood. The provider workshop was on Hands-On Hypnosis, my fusion of hypnosis and Reiki into a powerfully synthesized mind-body therapy. A cornerstone method in my practice, the training would foreshadow the value of this technique for those suffering on the other side of the globe.

There was suddenness to my decision to go to India. Many were confused by this rapid transition of focus from Guatemala to India. Were there not already plenty of relief workers on site? I spent much time explaining the drive behind my decision, in many cases to those who did not understand the Guatemala mission in the first place; they merely questioned the mercurial aspect of the change.

I did not know what to expect myself, only that in my heart it seemed the right thing to do and the portal of opportunity had opened and beckoned me. There persisted an eerie sense of imminent danger; with excitement and dread I packed my bags, wondering at times if I would return from this fanciful endeavor.

I had received a call from a stranger who was told of our trip by a friend. She reported that she had been to India fifteen times to work with Mother Teresa. She diligently directed me to take the food I would need for the trip in my luggage, along with a couple of bottles of liquor to bribe the Indian customs guards. This counsel was quickly dismissed. I told her of the nature of my mission, using hands-on, hypnosis-based trauma recovery methods to help those who were tsunami-affected. She hastily began to lambast me, saying "only Jesus can touch people and heal them. Who do you think you are? You are not Jesus."

This was not an entirely unfamiliar response to the work, though it had never been so blunt. Ten years into using hypnosis to help people alleviate their pain and suffering, there seemed to be a persistent barricade of incredulity around the whole notion. I found myself constantly clarifying to both the medical and lay community that what I offered was not some form of fraudulent hucksterism. The notion of healing through touch was often dismissed as even more bizarre and outlandish.

These responses always bewildered me. Since childhood I have had a fascination with "the power of the mind". In the early '70s, the television show *Kung Fu* opened with a scene of David Carradine placing his forearms against a glowing brazier to apply the Shaolin dragon brand. My brothers and I thought this a true testament to the power of mind, so we regularly challenged one another to endurance feats requiring physical and mental strength. By the time Uri Geller was demonstrating the passing of wires through his forearms, we were all devotees to this mystique.

My father first introduced the idea of hypnosis during a family dinner in 1972. A Marine, he had witnessed a hypnosis demonstration on base that day and reported not on silly actions, but on the specific nature of the mind to follow instruction and produce suggested outcomes. The fascination of that report formed a foundation for all the study I would later pursue.

Although I would continue to investigate the phenomena of consciousness in spiritual and performance dimensions, it would be over twenty years from that dinner to my formal study and practice of hypnosis. I was astounded to learn the breadth of its application. I learned that hypnosis and its pre-cursor Mesmerism were the first surgical anesthesia methods. They were used decades before chloroform and ether and without adverse, even fatal effects on the patient. I learned that hypnosis was also used in the United Sates as early as the Civil War, not only to help with treatment of battlefield injuries, but also to help resolve the distress of soldiers traumatized by war. This application would continue throughout all American wars to help with the ever-changing condition known as "shell shock", "combat fatigue", and "post-traumatic stress disorder". It was the use of hypnosis in the treatment of burns and the potential to strengthen immunity that truly stirred my mind to find a way to help the suffering.

I was equally dumbfounded by the dismissal of the healing power of touch. Although physical contact is almost instinctive in providing comfort, many still regarded its use as a therapeutic method as the stuff of storybooks. Oddly, in the context of the telephone conversation, it was actually my experience in Pentecostal Christianity that first informed my practice of healing through the "laying on of hands". Only later would I learn formal techniques and systems such as Reiki that carried this "healing virtue" from the sanctuary to the treatment room. It was, in all honesty, the enduring legacy of Jesus Christ that informed my odyssey to help others through the reassurance of compassionate touch and encouraging words.

She had, however, truly broken through with the critical question of "who do you think you are?" There is no greater way to "put a person back in their place" than to challenge them with this question. Underlying insecurities and inadequacies could always be called forward with this question. I had been confronted in similar ways repeatedly in the past, even in my own mind. Perhaps there was already someone more highly qualified than myself. I may only be intruding into the domain of true professionals with long-established agencies better equipped to work in disaster zones. These nagging concerns had challenged every step forward in planning.

This question, however, was one that I could already confidently answer. I knew my capability in the face of great physical and emotional challenge, not only for myself, but for hundreds of others I had already helped. I knew my ability to provide simple, yet highly effective interventions for those managing the complexity of living and dying with AIDS. I knew my ability to help individuals in writhing pain from decades of chronic suffering, roadside emergencies, and even hospitalization. I knew my ability to help persons with the most challenging pain problems for which strong medicines offered little relief.

I had asked myself the same question the first day I sought to help a person who was quadriplegic from spinal cord injury and, though unable to move from the neck down, was in burning pain that morphine only reduced from a level of 9 to 8.5. I answered that question by watching this same person, and several others in similar condition, virtually make the pain disappear. I knew my ability to help those I had worked with for ten years overcome lifetimes of distress and dismay. I had, years earlier, leaned closely to whisper into the ear of a client in the quiet domain of hypnotic trance "Remember who you are." It had become a mantra of self-possession, the essential elixir of accomplishment.

I did not know with certainty that I could help those suffering from devastation on the other side of the planet. I did have confidence that if anyone could, I could.

I did not share this thought with my challenger. Despite my instinct to simply hang up the phone, I continued to listen as she further pronounced that I would die from the diseases I would encounter in India. I held the phone, feeling as though I was hearing curses placed upon me a cackling witch, but I have learned to listen for wisdom, even in madness. I took the call as a serious warning to guard my health in this unknown and hazardous place. These concerns were compounded when a friend who was in India during the tsunami had to return to the states for treatment from a bite from the disfiguring elephantiasis-causing fly.

As I continued to endure her vitriol, suddenly the jewel emerged: "…just remember, you are walking on the sacred ground of the poor." Those words resonated deeply within me and set my compass bearing for the mission. Our organization, First Medicines, was founded on the principle of developing internal, personal capabilities through our simple combined methods. Respect for the individual and what they bring is considered paramount. When I heard this statement, it framed the manner of this dynamic in my mind. I was going to be a guest and servant; whatever I brought in the way of benefits was solely a gift for those I would serve.

This philosophy of identifying and strengthening abilities already present in the population also led to continuous contributions to the understanding and application of the work. The HIV/AIDS and spinal cord injury populations had guided me to tailor methods to their presenting needs and helped me understand the value of trauma recovery in health management. The culture of Guatemala had informed the structure of the organization. I expected the people of India to also both receive benefit and add greater dimension to First Medicines.

A few days after the call, Jim and I met to give each other bodywork treatments. During my treatment from Jim, a remarkable thing happened. I knew that we would visit the carved stone temples of Mamallapuram, so I conducted a little research into the area, complete with review of many photos. These images began to inform a vision during my treatment.

In my vision, I was standing on a shore looking out at the rolling waves. Jim had suggested that I be mindful of all the people who were supporting me in the mission. I sensed this grand company standing behind me. I felt their individual and group presence. As I turned to look behind me, the image of the throng was transformed into a massive stone wall, similar to those I had seen in the photos. The stones began to move, and from them emerged a colossal beast made up of the huge grey rough-hewn stones. He rose up, standing stories high with muscular human legs, torso, and arms, yet the head of a bull-like beast with great horns. Smoke billowed from his nostrils as he approached me. I was not afraid, only awed. As he drew near, he extended his closed hand toward me, opened it, and looking directly into my eyes, bellowed "I give you my strength." I felt my whole being swell with this sense of power. My confidence in the mission surged. I opened my eyes, ready to go.

At ten o'clock in the morning of February 1st, Lenise dropped me off in front of the Tom Bradley International Terminal at Los Angeles International Airport. Mitta was waiting there with Mike Saul, her boyfriend. After our strained goodbyes, I watched Lenise drive off as I dragged my bag over the curb and onto the sidewalk. Mitta and I carried and pulled our luggage, one duffel bag and one backpack each, into the terminal and surrendered the larger bags to the security inspectors. We traveled around the corner, stepped up to the counter, and surrendered ourselves into the competent, caring hands of the crew at Singapore Airlines.

The flight was long but comfortable. I have always enjoyed flying, especially the high view of the passing landscape from the plane window. To my good fortune I was able to view, thirty thousand feet below, the snowy peaks of Alaska's Aleutian Islands jutting up from the sea. The dramatic contrast from sea to snow-capped ranges captured my imagination.

I had never traveled to Asia, so even the plane change in Tokyo was an adventure. In the terminal I encountered a man in a University of Oklahoma sweatshirt. En route to Dallas, he was a resident of Oklahoma City and lived near the neighborhood Lenise and I had spent much of the previous year while caring for her father. To my comfort, even though on the far side of the Pacific, I still encountered travelers from a familiar place.

We arrived in Singapore late that night and were ferried to a hotel for a sleepover before catching the flight to India the following evening. While in Singapore, we fulfilled a friend's mandate to enjoy a Singapore Sling at its birthplace, the Long Bar at Raffles Hotel. While there, a parade of individuals who appeared to be restaurant workers marched to the bar and assembled themselves before a bartender who began to display the utensils of his craft. I stepped to the bar and enjoyed a lesson in making the Sling while its sweet flavor still rested on my palate. After touring the city throughout the afternoon on a special bus, we rendezvoused with our luggage at the hotel and caught the bus to the airport.

The flight to Chennai was pleasant as well. We met a wonderful gentleman from New Delhi who was flying to see his family whom he had not been with for several years. Having traveled to many lands in the previous three years, I became attuned to the demographic on different planes, based on their origin and destination. I had noted the dramatic shift on this India-bound flight. The LA/International-styled group that I had flown to Singapore with had transformed into a mostly Indian group.

The transformation of the society I traveled with became a hint of the changes I would encounter at the next airport. We landed at the Chennai (formerly Madras) airport on schedule. As we traveled up the walkway, I smelled the familiar high-humidity mustiness I had also experienced in Singapore. As we entered the airport itself, I felt as though I had crossed a time threshold. Where the Singapore airport was modern and pristine, complete with armed security forces drilling at midnight, the Chennai airport seemed to have been built in the 1950's. It had tile mosaics on the walls reminiscent of the same era junior high school I had attended. Where previously we had stood in line at the immigration desk before glass and steel, here we queued up before an archaic bag-screening machine and were waved through by officers wearing uniforms that were somewhat less than starched and pressed. The baggage carousel also seemed from another time, but seemed to function well. I wondered if all the modern updates of my world were really that necessary.

We retrieved our bags and exited the claim area. Throngs of greeters lined the barriers as we walked from the internal reception area of the terminal into the cool, yet balmy Chennai night. There, front and center, was the placard held by our own greeter. I recognized him from the photos I had been shown by Jim in LA. With him was a friend who had joined him to help us with bags and the driver of the car he had hired for our hotel transit. We took a couple of quick arrival photos, then loaded into the Toyota Land Cruiser, safe from the lightly falling rain, home for now in India.

3

Dhamodharan's Village

Narayanan Dhamodharan resided in Srinivasapuram, a small coastal village on the outskirts of Chennai. Chennai was formerly known as Madras and is the capitol of the southern Indian state Tamil Nadu. Nestled between the districts of Mandaveli and Gandhi Nagar, with a population of approximately two thousand, this tranquil community of "Srini" is built around the single paved road that runs along its coastal facing. Small alleyways flow inland from the quarter-mile stretch of road to another wide walking-path like road. Similar alleyways flow from the seaward side through a series of dwellings that front the beach, opening up to the sand, beach, and the sea beyond.

Under normal circumstances, the beach is filled with fishing boats of a variety of styles, from twenty-five-foot fiberglass boats to hewn-beam kattumarams. The principle industry of the community is fishing. The men fish the sea with their boats and the women sell the fish in the market. Other small support services such as tiny booth-like markets, a butcher shop, a tailor, plus a "wine-shop" bar make up the small enclave that is also served by a beautiful large temple and several small ones. The children fly kites on the beach and chase balls in the street while by day and night neighbors sit outside their homes, enjoying one another's company.

On the morning of December 26, Dhamodharan was visiting a friend about one hour's journey by bus from his home. He received a call from a friend who told him a catastrophe had taken place; he must return at once. When he got within one-half hour from his home, he saw crowds of people walking and mayhem in the street. People were moving like a single mass, fleeing in a panic.

By the time he reached his village, the scene had become even more distressing. People were wandering the streets aimlessly in a daze. Stripped nude by the waves, they roamed like zombies. Rising above the sound of the suffering crowd was a wail that took on a life of its own, cries of grief and names called out despairingly.

Dhamodharan arrived at his apartment only yards from the sand to find his family gone, along with all of their possessions. Upturned appliances littered the wasteland that was previously his home. He ran calling into the chaos, seeking his family in the throng. It was almost nightfall when he found them. They were huddled together on a sidewalk near the entrance to the village. They had been warned of the wave and ran to the upper floor of the apartment building as the surge decimated their own dwelling. With only the soaked clothes on their bodies, they fled during an abatement of the water. Shivering against the cold of the approaching night, his parents, sisters, aunt, nephews and niece had all survived, and now they clung only to one another.

Sometime during the cold of the night, as the family held each other close to stay warm, a stranger arrived and gave them a blanket. This gift from an unknown friend became their only barrier against the cruel circumstances they endured. Homeless and without possessions, bewildered like so many others, they operated from their small square of concrete to recover any remnants from their ruined home and rebuild their lives.

It was during these first of twelve days spent living on the sidewalk that Dhamodharan's concerns moved beyond just those of his family, but also to the plight of the entire village. In this devastation, he began to see a greater need than rice and plastic tarps. Rebuilding the village would also require rebuilding the villagers, helping to restore their individual capabilities, and empowering them to reach for something more. Aware of benefits he had received through a good education, particularly learning English and completing his Masters Degree, he now dreamed of providing similar opportunities to the children of his village. He knew he could not do it on his own; he decided to ask for help from his "Uncle" in America, Jim Rudolph.

Through the generosity of many friends, Jim was able to raise funds to help Dhamodharan and his family with food, clothing, and shelter. Dhamodharan then turned his focus to the children of the village. Because they too had lost all of their clothing and possessions, he designed a project to provide school uniforms for all of the children so they could return to their studies with dignity. He canvassed the village to enroll all in need and assess individual styles and sizes. Involving the entire family and others in the project, they then assembled the uniforms and distributed them to the village children.

Encouraged by the good results obtained through the school uniform project, Dhamodharan began to look toward other ways to help his village. He was encouraged when "Jim Uncle" told him that a teacher from the United States would come to help those who had been emotionally distressed by the tsunami. He began to consider how to develop training opportunities for those in the village, though he had little information on the exact method of training and therapy that would be offered. He considered that he may even be able to use this help to reach beyond his village, to those in other nearby villages who might be suffering. With diligence, he undertook the assignment and made the necessary arrangements for lodging and transportation. Then, he met Mr. Timothy Trujillo and Mitta at the airport.

4

Talking to Water

We zipped through the rain-soaked Chennai traffic and I quickly realized that road rules were not the same in India as in America. Lines and lanes have little meaning. We rushed up behind a truck, staring down the menacingly grinning face painted on the rear transaxle of the truck, as motorcycles scooted between and around us.

Dhamodharan and I discussed plans along the way. He made a full report of all the arrangements he had made and informed us of his eagerness to realize the success of our project. He informed us that his friend Vijay, who had carried our bags and now sat in the front seat, was also excited to help out. It was suggested that since the village was on the way to the hotel, if desired, we could stop and see some of the effects of the tsunami on the village.

We drove down the narrow road that turned right to lead down some one-fourth of a mile along the beach, the main road of the village. We stopped not far down the road and climbed out of the Land Cruiser. There was a smell of stale seawater in the air as we walked down a narrow pathway between small mud-brick buildings that soon opened out onto a beach. At the edge of the sand, was a pile of bricks and wood and palm fronds. "Here," said Dhamodharan, "is Vijay's house."

We looked at the pile of broken wood and masonry, highly visible in the night, and offered our condolences to Vijay. Now, tsunami was no longer an idea or a news report, but an enduring personal tragedy of a friend.

"I'd like to go down and talk to the water." I told Dhamodharan. We headed across the sand toward the surf.

"You know the language of water?" Dhamodharan said, as we walked to meet the tide.

I stood on the water's edge, drinking in the air and the environment, feeling a sense of place and presence. The vision from my time with Jim was still strong in my mind and a part of me wanted to record and catalog this environment to match it with that of my imagination. I stood and let the waves roll, synching to their rhythm. I stepped down to the water and scooped a bit in my hands, then brought it toward my face. I stood again, and in my stillness, spoke in the silence of my thoughts to the sea.

We turned to head to the vehicle. Each step now seemed a bit more planted and present. I felt at once at home, but in a solemn space where great hardship had taken place. We arrived at the vehicle, now turned about, and headed for the hotel.

Nearing midnight, yet uncertain of my own actual physical time clock, we settled into our rooms at the MGM Grand Hotel of Chennai. Dhamodharan gave me maps of Chennai and Tamil Nadu, set our meeting time for the morning, and offered "good sleep and good dreams."

I spent a little time unpacking and making notes in my journal before I retired for the night, happy to be settled in after the long journey and filled with anticipation for the next day's adventures.

I awoke at about eight o'clock, arose feeling well-rested, and opened the drapes to allow the outside light into the room. Crows were cackling a symphony, punctuated by the constant beeping of horns on the street below. I spent some time in meditation to center myself and be present to this new world, and then went to the door to find, delivered there, the English-language newspaper.

The hotel desk called the room and asked if I wanted coffee. They brought a carafe filled with coffee mixed with cream. I sent it back and requested coffee with no cream. When they brought the carafe back, they had simply emptied the coffee and refilled it with black coffee that was now speckled with cream droplets. My stomach turned and I remembered a warning from Jim regarding milk products, so I denied myself the coffee in hopes of preserving my health. What I had tried unsuccessfully to do for two years, quit coffee, I now did in a moment thanks to the right motivation.

I ate my simple breakfast of peanut butter on granola bars in my room then went down to the street for a walk. After Mitta returned from her own stroll to the beach a few blocks away, we met for a more robust breakfast in the hotel restaurant as we waited for Dhamodharan's arrival.

We agreed to a light schedule in order to acclimate, taking care of some shopping and other errands before meeting Dhamodharan's family for dinner in the evening. Vijay waited outside the hotel with the two-wheelers (motorcycles) while we made our arrangements. Soon another friend, Basker, arrived driving an autorickshaw, our transportation for the day and what would become a very familiar vehicle during our stay.

The autorickshaw, a ubiquitous sight in India, is a small three-wheeled vehicle with a canvass top. It is well-suited for two passengers, but more can be crowded in, as is commonly necessary. It is driven with handlebars, rather than a steering wheel and a lever that is pulled to start it. It commonly bears a rubber-bulb bicycle horn, a critical instrument for effective driving. Its two-stroke motor seems powerful enough to carry any load, but belches white smoke when aged or under strain. Another appealing feature is that its light weight makes it easy to lift or roll onto its side for repairs or push here or there, particularly as it has no reverse gear. In Chennai, the most common color combination is a yellow body with a black top.

We loaded into the "auto", three in the back with Vijay up front with Basker, and headed off to Spencer Plaza for shopping. We scurried through the labyrinthine mall like rats after cheese, found many of our desired goods, and finished the shopping spree with a wrapped potato samosa from a snack stand before dashing off to our next errand.

I was happy to find a wonderful pair of Bata sandals at a special shop down the road, outside of which the street vendors had a delirious time selling us trinkets from their small tarp-on-the-ground shop. A familiar site at various locations, these street vendors would come to equip us with many precious souvenirs. We would learn, however, that they were a very unreliable source for cheap electronics that had the unpleasant feature of exploding when plugged into the wall.

After a bit more shopping, we stopped at a small restaurant for lunch. We entered the noisy cafeteria-styled seating area and found a table that would accommodate us. On the wall was a small sink over which was written the word "wash". We took our turns washing our hands, particularly as we had learned that our right hand would be our eating utensil. We enjoyed a moderate lunch of breads and curries and finished with a sweet ice cream delight. Following this late afternoon treat, we headed back to the hotel to prepare for our first visit with Dhamodharan's family.

5

Grass Mat Diplomacy

Riding on the two-wheelers, we danced, leaning against the wind we created as we sped through the Chennai night traffic on our way to Srinivasapuram. Vijay and Dhamodharan our "charioteers", we jetted toward our destination, Dhamodharan's former home. His family had gathered to welcome us. We brought simple gifts of chocolate and other treats. As we dismounted, a flurry of excitement surrounded the bikes as the local children gathered to meet the foreigners.

We shook hands with many and exchanged names with a few before walking down the narrow pathway and into the small two-room apartment that had been the family's previous home. As we passed through the door, we were met with enthusiasm and warmth. We exchanged cordial greetings that included the Tamil manner of placing palms together at chest level in prayer position and saying "Vanakam" or "God Bless You". We also demonstrated our custom of greeting, the handshake and the hug. Most of Dhamodharan's extended family was in attendance: his mother and father, two aunts and an uncle, his three sisters, plus two nephews and niece.

As we walked through the door, Dhamodharan's father, Narayanan, walked to the wall and began to point out the waterline stain that was about six feet up the wall and another that was about a foot below it. Speaking in Tamil with pantomime gestures, he explained how the water had come in twice to those levels, causing everything in the house to become waterborne. Dhamodharan translated as the rest of the family joined in to show how they had run out of the room and up the stairs to the second floor. They all conveyed their excitement at once, relating the drama of their ordeal, while Dhamodharan continued to translate one thread of the tale after the other.

A grass mat was brought from the other room and laid down on the floor and two plastic patio-styled chairs were brought out and placed on it. Narayanan gestured for us to sit; we obligingly took our places. Suddenly, with one voice, the entire family began to celebrate "Jim Uncle", their familiar name for Jim Rudolph. A black and white photograph of Jim was brought from the other room, shown to us, and then properly displayed in the room where we were sitting. Jim was not just a family member and patron. They honored him with the respect due a deity, an honor I would learn was well-founded. I also learned that the title "Uncle" means any family relationship or kin. It is also used for one who is like a family member.

Someone said "cold drinks!" and soon two cups of cold and sparkling orange soda were brought out. We sipped on the sodas as we accepted their further hospitality to prepare food for us. They reassured us that Jim Uncle had given them special instructions on what foods would be good to keep our stomachs safe. Jim had cautioned Mitta and I about eating food prepared in the villages, as certain bacteria and parasites that the locals had adapted to could make us very ill, particularly those in milk products.

As we sat and enjoyed the cavalcade of family tales, the eldest of Dhamodharan's nephews, Deepash, was brought before me. About six, he stood looking into my face with his dark and innocent eyes. He had the presence of a morning dove, calm, yet quivering. He was a bit shy to talk, but when I took his palm and read the lines in it for him, he took great interest. Following the indications in his hand, I asked if he had good dreams. He said yes, that he greatly enjoyed experiences that he had while dreaming. I told him that he should begin to write down these dream stories. He consented and his mother and grandmother both thought it a good idea.

Next, I was presented with Jodash, the two-year old nephew who was introduced as a "very dangerous guy". Within moments, observing his sudden wrestling tirade, I understood their meaning. We learned more of the family's affairs as we were directed to sit on the floor where, upon another mat, a tray of food and beverage was arranged. We took our places and began to enjoy the meal. I pronounced the food "DEE-licious," which amused Dhamodharan's sister with its down-home drawl.

We sat visiting for a couple of hours. We enjoyed the meal of tomato sandwiches, rice, and especially the bananas served as desert to "help cool the body." We spoke of school interests and aspects of our lives in America, then turned our conversation to the work that we had come to do. When I was asked about my adjustments to the time change, I reported that I had used my mind to reset my body's clock to India time. I explained my hypnotic method of breath control and relaxation and "talking to the body." Saraswathy, the youngest of the sisters, sat upright and exclaimed "yoga!" My uncertainty regarding explanation and acceptance of our methods was instantly allayed. I had considered couching the method as a kind of yoga, but she had spontaneously confirmed my analogy.

During this time, we had stretched out our legs on the floor in order to be more comfortable. Saraswathy reached across and grabbed my long middle toe in her fingers and, giving it a yank, sent a crackling down my foot. She then proceeded to do the same for each toe and followed it up with a foot and leg massage, repeating the same on the other foot and leg. Meanwhile Dhamodharan's other sister, Subathra, began to care for Mitta in a similar manner, eventually producing polish to groom her nails.

We enjoyed our time together for the remainder of the evening, accepting their invitation to come for dinner each night that our work did not keep us away. While departing, we were introduced to Vijay's family members as we strode back down the pathway, climbed aboard the two-wheelers, and galloped back to the hotel.

6

The Children of Muttukadu

We had made arrangements to visit the ancient temple site, Mamallapuram, about one hour's drive south of Chennai. Dhamodharan hired a driver and car, another Toyota Land Cruiser. Vijay and Basker joined us for the trip. We drove south out of Chennai, through Adyar and other small communities, or Nagars, eventually seeing the congested shops lining the roadway give way to open fields. Along the way, we stopped at a small market for water and snacks. While standing by the roadside, I was compelled to yield to a cow walking down the same road shoulder, on her way to what I am certain was an important engagement. I asked Dhamu why she was walking freely with no apparent owner or identification. He explained that was the way of cows and the owner knew well of her location. I wanted to pet the cow, as she seemed so docile, but was warned that calamity would come upon me if I touched another man's cow.

We passed a beachfront amusement park, MGM Dizzy World, whose inviting façade seemed like any other park I had seen in the US, though a little less glitzy. Just beyond the amusement park, the driver turned down a dirt road and drove about one fourth of a mile to a small village on the beach. We drove down a small dirt road that fronted the beach as Dhamodharan turned to me to say, "This is a village that was very tsunami-affected, the people forced to go away."

The driver stopped. We got out of the vehicle and walked about on the silent road. We could see that the huts and small block houses that faced the beach had been damaged. Beyond them, toward the beach, slabs of concrete house foundations were jostled and jutting upward, torn from their sandy moorings. A few damaged boats lay scattered on the beach. As we stood taking in the environment, two elderly women came walking toward us on the dusty road, one hand outwardly stretched as the other moved from covering the stomach to pressing clustered fingers to the lips. This gesture I immediately understood to mean "I'm hungry, please give me some food." I later learned it also meant "Please give me some money so I can buy some food." Also, in its shorter version of fingers to lips meant "Please, two rupees for tea." This, one of the most valuable communications I would learn.

Dhamodharan had given us careful instructions not to give away any rupees without first checking with him. Reluctantly I refused to give money to the women, but instead referred them to Dhamodharan who, after visiting with them for a few minutes, requested that I give them twenty rupees and a banana each.

We were joined by a couple of the village men, traditionally attired in tee shirt and lungi, a skirt-like piece of fabric worn long or folded short, particularly while working. They were accompanied by Basker, who was uncle to one of the men. After our greetings, we were taken on a tour of the village, beginning on the beach. Basker's uncle took us into his house, one of those fronting the beach. As we walked through the door, he stepped to the wall and pointed to the familiar waterline mark, here about four feet high. We walked through the empty house to an open door facing the sea. He pointed out the door and said a large patio area had been washed away, leaving only the sand, palm fronds, and a broken, tilting slab of concrete.

We walked outside and down the road, viewing similarly decimated homes along the way. At the end of the road, there was a drop to an inlet. Along its banks were palm trees that had been toppled when the tsunami crashed by, leaving eight foot tall root balls protruding from the sand. We clambered down the embankment to face large piles of nets, twisted and tangled into massive wads and peppered with other debris. Dhamodharan pointed across the inlet, some seventy-five yards, and said "Here stood a temple that was completely washed away; the god was taken out to sea, gone."

We walked to the site and now in its place were only a few stacked bricks and some recent offerings. Around the makeshift altar was open space, scoured clean by the wave. We crossed the dry inlet back to the homes and walked down a small promenade, faced on each side by damaged and abandoned houses. Scattered here and there remained debris from the lives that formerly occupied the village: boat motors, schoolbooks, clothing, and furniture, all soaked and rotting in piles of other remnants such as bricks and wood. Between two homes the severed bow of a fishing boat was wedged amongst other castaway flotsam. A haunting silence echoed through the alleys and walkways as we made our way back to the car.

When we arrived at the car, several villagers greeted us, seeking a ride. As many as could be fit were crowded into the back of the Toyota Cruiser and we were off. About one mile down the highway a field of brightly colored tents became visible on the seaward side of the road. We turned onto a dirt path and parked beneath two great shade trees, under which many villagers were also taking refuge from the midday heat.

I stepped out of the car and a small boy arose from his mat, extended his hand, pointed to his chest, and said "Sathish."

I repeated the name, and then mimicked his own gesture, saying "Timothy."

"Ah, Timotee," he responded.

The others climbed out of the vehicle, including our passengers, and we followed our guide Sathish up the dirt path to the tent camp. Along the path, I bent down and recovered a broken marble, discarded and covered in the sand. We walked further into the maze of tents constructed of tarpaulins colored green and blue and orange. In front of one of the tents, a young woman sat before a smoldering terracotta firepot. Atop the firepot a steel pot steeped, cooking the midday meal. Her infant child was playing nearby in the narrow "yard" that separated the fronts of the tents. Our parade through camp continued down the narrow walkways between the tents, stepping over ties and around stakes along the way.

We arrived at a tent on the far side of the camp, beyond which were open fields sweeping down the quarter-mile or less to the sea. Across from the tents were about four small timber hut frames, skeletons of developing dwellings. From within one of the tents, a gentleman emerged, dressed like the other fishermen in a lungi, but wearing it long, with a more formal button-up shirt with collar. His name was Ramalinga, a key village leader who, though not tall, carried himself with the stature of a giant. Dhamodharan explained to Ramalinga the work that we had come to do.

We were paraded on to a few other tents where we were introduced to more of Basker's relations and the mother of Vijay's soon-to-be wife. We walked out of the encampment to the group of villagers sitting under the tree. Ramalinga polled the villagers to learn of any still suffering from injury or loss from the tsunami, any who were still "tsunami-affected".

A gentleman who had been with us in the village earlier approached us to say that his son had been disturbed in his mind since the tsunami.

He said that all he wanted to do was throw stones. I requested to be taken to the boy.

We followed a path toward a nearby structure that had been converted into an improvised schoolhouse. Some children playing in the "schoolyard" greeted us as we passed by toward the preschool area. A small boy, about four, was brought out of the room where around thirty little children were napping on mats, supervised by their teachers. The boy's father compelled him to move toward me, though he clung tightly to his father's leg, weeping with fear. I placed my hand on the boy's shoulder. He recoiled a little and then yielded, all the while clinging more tightly to his father's leg.

The father told us that during the tsunami all in the village were running frantically from the waves. The desperate flight was filled with chaos and screams of despair. His distress rising above his threshold of coping or understanding, the little boy collapsed and fell while running and began a fit of screaming. After being scooped up and carried to safety, he continued to shudder uncontrollably. In time, the shaking settled down, but the frown, weepy eyes, jutted lower lip, and fragile, hostile temperament remained.

As Dhamodharan interpreted, I told the father that his son's heart had been very disturbed by the fear that he had experienced. I demonstrated the gentle rocking technique I was using to calm the boy, very subtly moving my hand while resting on the shoulder. I told the father that it may take a long period of time for his son to recover, but that he should practice this technique to settle him when he was in a fit and that he should hold the boy closely each day and tell him that he is loved and safe with his family.

In my further effort to connect with the boy, I produced my flute from my backpack and began to play a few notes. He shrank back against his father's leg but kept his eyes on me as I played. Several of the children who had gathered around stood with amused gazes at the strange flute, a Native American flute, and the even stranger song it produced.

A small girl was brought forward. Three years old, her name was Monika. Her father tried to explain that there was a problem with her face but I could see no wound or bruising. Monika opened her mouth, exposing some teeth, but when I inspected them I saw no irregularities. I then noticed that only one side of her mouth was opening to expose the teeth and when I made a few faces for her to mimic, I realized that the right side of her face was paralyzed.

I placed my hands on each cheek and began to give her Reiki treatment. She looked up at me, so patiently enduring our inspection and intervention, accepting our efforts to help her. I took her little hands and held them to her own cheeks, placing my hands on top of hers. We sat for a few minutes that way, with no words. Then I placed my hands on my own cheeks to compel her to keep her hands on her own for a while. All this time, I was letting her father know to give her this very type of treatment daily. Her father reassured us that he would give Monika the treatments and was thankful that he had some way to help.

Dhamodharan spoke with the teachers regarding their critical educational needs. They told him that the little ones needed slates to practice their letters. We were given a count and told them we would return with the necessary materials.

By now the driver had arrived at the schoolyard. I packed my flute away and Vijay took the bag, carrying it gleefully back to the car. The spirit of the children's gentle kindness with us, we headed to Mamallapuram.

7

Mamallapuram

The roadway rolled before us with cinematic splendor, framed on either side by open fields, rural temples, and small tent encampments of other villages displaced by the tsunami. Tamil music blared from the stereo as we all swayed with the maneuvering vehicle, roaming our gaze from scenery to one another, rapt by the mystique of coastal South India. The intrigue of the foreign landscape was matched only by the sense of mystery I had experienced since arriving, in both my waking thoughts and dreams.

During the previous night, I had had a very strange, vivid dream. In my dream, I was lecturing to a group of students when the bell rang, releasing the class. Most students went their way, but a few stayed for last questions and comments. When finished, I exited the classroom and walked outdoors. I had made a plan to meet a friend at his place, which was a short walk from the school. As I walked down the sidewalk, I began to increase my pace, then dropped my hands to the ground and began to run on all four limbs like a jaguar. I pranced with grace down the sidewalk, watching driveways and lawns pass by. Soon, I began to run with my left leg extended straight out behind me in the air as only my right leg and arms maintained my steady gallop.

People came and went in their driveways as I felt the concrete sidewalk rolling by beneath my hands. A small boy pointed to me and made comments to his father at the strange way I was running, particularly with my leg flagging like the backside of a white-tailed deer. I came upon a house with a hedged fence encircling the front yard. I scrambled over the fence and, once in the yard, began to search for the path out. An old man stepped onto the front porch and motioned to a spot in the hedge on the opposite side of the yard. I leapt upon a barrel, then sprang over the hedge and continued on my way.

After panting and prancing like a predator with nose to the wind, I arrived at my destination. I entered my friend's small apartment, stood upright, like a were-jaguar returning to human form, and walked across the room to look out a window from which I could see a small garden plot in the yard. My friend entered the room and greeted me. As he passed by and entered the kitchen to take a call, I felt a tickling on my back. I brushed myself and observed a large winged insect, nearly a foot long, fall to the ground and scramble away. I awakened with the strangest sense of presence, pressing fingers to palms where I seemingly had paw pads only moments before. India, I thought, had captured my dream world as well.

We arrived at Mamallapuram and drove directly to the large carving known as "Arjuna's Penance", a forty foot high carved stone wall relief representing a scene from the classic Hindu tale, Mahabharata. In the research that I did when learning that I would visit this site, I saw images of this very carving. Now, standing before its larger-than-imagined daunting scale, I basked in the sense of being present in a spot only known to me from a picture book. I truly was in this faraway place; my hopes and dreams had become my reality.

A street vendor lost no time catching the arriving foreigners with his small basket of carved works, treasures he insisted we purchase for a king's ransom. Dhamodharan intervened and, after some haggling in a foreign tongue with familiar tones, we swapped rupees for trinkets and continued on our way. The site is a rambling array of small cave temples carved into massive granite stones strewn along an outcropping between the coast and a natural harbor. A seaport since ancient times, the tradition of carving the temples and reliefs dates to about 700 A.D.

As Dhamodharan and the guys went for food, Mitta and I continued to investigate the various carvings. A young guide approached us and began to explain the different sites, cleverly attempting to lead us to a carving shop to purchase more gifts. With some effort, we persuaded him that we would not shop and were left on our way.

We climbed to the high point, where what appeared to be a temple was carved from a protruding stone. Another guide met us by the site and informed us it was a lighthouse from ancient times, a large carved stone base rising ten feet, atop which a bonfire was ignited, giving light for vessels at sea. From this high spot, I heard a persistent sound rising from the valley below, the steady clinking of hammer and chisel upon stone. A symphony of stone carvers' strikes echoed throughout the valley and drifted up the hill, carrying my imagination to the distant reaches of time when the same sounds, centuries earlier, created the sites we were viewing. A large monkey, true native of the area and unperturbed by our presence, sauntered along the pipe guardrail and literally leapt over my head to scramble to the top of the lighthouse, somehow expressing his ownership of the site.

Our new guide was grand. He gave us a wondrous history lesson and clear explanations of the scenes in the various carvings. We stepped into an elaborate cave with elegantly carved columns, part of the original stone. On one wall I saw a giant carved relief of a battle scene. One of the figures in the scene was very similar to the stone beast I had seen in my vision. I was perplexed by this at first. I knew enough of the stories and had seen enough images to know that this was the bad guy. Why would he give his power to support our project? I remembered being told that in many of the battles between gods and demons, when the demon was defeated, it surrendered its power to the god. Willingly, it seemed, the beast was surrendering something of himself for the people of India.

On the adjacent wall was a carving of the great god Vishnu, sleeping on his serpent-hooded bed. Standing in the remarkably crafted sacred space, opening out past the columns to a sunny valley, I felt myself drifting in the dream of the sleeping god.

A real pro, the guide had not yet mentioned the shop that he would ultimately seek to direct us toward after our "tour". Beating him to his punch, I promised that due to his exquisite guidance, I would visit his carving shop and make a purchase after reconnecting with our "negotiators". We followed the path from the lighthouse to the carving shop to preview his wares, then walked along the dirt roadway back to our rendezvous spot. Along either side of the narrow road were stone-carving shops from which the persistent clinking rang as stone dust drifted into the street like a rolling fog.

We reached our rendezvous point and the others could not be found. Mitta began to swoon from the heat and insisted on finding a drink. I, too, began to feel the effects of the sun, the heat and humidity, and the general disorientation of time and place. Soon Dhamu and the others appeared, their bellies filled, and delivered us to an "American Hotel" where we could get food that would be safe for us to eat.

After reviving ourselves with some fresh and familiar food, we set out for the Shore Temple. We approached what was a much more commercial attraction with booths and vendors offering treasured trinkets, talismans of the visit to this noble shrine. With some negotiations and complaints that westerners paid a higher rate than locals, we acquiesced, at the counsel of Dhamu, and happily gave our rupees to behold the ancient masterworks.

As we passed the gate, we were approached by a rather eloquently English-speaking local who offered to serve as our guide to the site, bringing his twenty years of experience. He had, in these two decades, learned well how to tell the story of the place and kept us engaged and informed through our tour of the spectacular temples built of massive granite blocks on the shore. Built on a stone escarpment, they seemed to rise from the sand then blossom into their ornately carved roofs, burnished by the winds of time. Piece by piece our guide explained the carvings and their depictions of events both known and unknown. He also knew which settings to best exploit for photos and quickly maneuvered through the operational challenges of my digital camera.

The sun was sliding low in the western sky as we exited the Shore Temple site en route to another carving site we wanted to see before dusk. As we passed through the gate, I noticed a fellow, about my age, with a group of others near the vendors. His hands were on the ground and he walked around, as it were, on all fours. His left leg, clearly affected by polio, stretched directly out behind him in the air. I felt, as the British say, "gob-smacked". He was exactly as I had been in my dream the previous night. A wave of profound mystery washed over me as I approached him to try to make some sense of the absolute strangeness of the event. I told him that I had dreamed that I was walking like him. He told me, through translation, that he thought that was a good thing, a good sign. I spent just a few moments with him, trying to wade through my bewilderment. I sensed that perhaps I had, in my dream, connected with the very soul of this place. I offered him a generous gift of rupees and departed with a sense of kindness and oneness.

The next site was equally engaging, the Pancha Rathas, small shrines to the brothers from the Mahabharata. They included a shrine to the beloved Drobadai, heroine of the tale. On the wall of one of the shrines, I recognized a carving of Shiva as male on one side and female on the other. I had seen such images, perhaps this one, in the videos of Joseph Campbell commenting on its depiction of the nature of dualism. Standing before it here was as equally awe-inspiring as my experience viewing the Rosetta Stone in the British Museum years earlier. During my moments of rapture, the guys purchased some small souvenir statues from a strolling vendor and made a gift of them to us and Jim Uncle.

We strolled from this site down the dusty streets we had visited earlier in the day as the fading light created a grey hew on the stone-carvers shops. We heard a commotion and came upon a group of boys bantering around a top spinning on the ground. They danced about the tiny "dervish" with skips and hops and shouts of glee. One boy stepped from the group, whipped a piece of string about the base of the spinner like a lariat and, with a flick, the top took flight from the ground and landed in his hand, still spinning. The challenge was on.

Another boy stepped forward, still winding the string about the base of his wooden charger, and with a confident pitch and pull, sent the top whistling to the ground. The child and juggler within me lurched like the top with the same vigor, my empty hands preventing me from entering the dance. I contented myself instead to lend my exuberance to the scene, joining the cluster as though this had been my destination all along.

I felt a tug at my arm. The light was fading and we still had to make a visit to our guide's shop. Reluctantly, I turned from my newfound pals and headed further down the street. Dhamodharan leaned in to comfort me "Uncle, I have sent Basker to purchase a top for your grandson."

As we approached the tiny shop, our guide greeted us with great kindness and promised to provide the best bargain for our faithfulness in returning. I stepped into what amounted to a small closet lined with shelves filled with arrays of different figures and objects carved from the local stone. As we shopped for our perfect treasure, the dust that hung in the shop, accumulating on the shelves for generations, suddenly sucked the breath from the very root of my lungs. My sinuses first itched then swelled from the insulting air, as the headache I had been holding at bay lurched into my head like an un-tethered beast. I felt faint, then nauseous. The light seemed to close around me as I urgently paid the shopkeeper for the small black Ganesha sculpture I had selected and stumbled toward the waiting car.

Panic seized me. The vice-like grip on my head and body sent me into a delirium. "No!" I thought. "Not at the very start. I refuse to become ill before our work here even begins." I pushed back against the grip of pain, gathered my focus, and began to tend to my breathing and employ other self-hypnotic pain relief methods. Thinking I may have picked up some food bug, Mitta produced a small bottle of grapefruit seed extract and put a few drops in a bottle of water then gave it to me to sip as she set to work with acupressure to my hand. Waves of chills and sweat overcame me as we rolled out of Mamallapuram toward Chennai, our taxi now more like an ambulance.

8

Strongbody

One hour later, as we reached the outskirts of Adyar, just south of Chennai, my head was beginning to clear. The shop lights were coming into clear focus and people became more than blurred blobs assaulting my field of vision. The relief of the passing of the storm and the reassurance within that I would live gave me an expansive sense. It felt like a first breath, a rebirth in which possibilities opened before me as immense potential already fulfilled in my imagination. Having faced and overcome the challenge, I felt restored, capable, and invincible. By the time we reached the hotel, I possessed the strength and outlook one feels at the beginning of the day.

We settled with our driver and headed up to the room for a brief recap with the group. In the elevator, Dhamodharan turned uneasily toward me in the tiny chamber and asked with respect and bewilderment "Uncle, I have every confidence in you, but I must have understanding in order to help you. Please tell me how this flute is going to help my people."

Clearly, he had had his own quandary during the day. After observing me produce the flute in the village to play for the children, he was trying to wade through his own mystery of the strangers from afar. He had been told we would bring abilities to help ease the suffering of his people. We had produced no medicines, no bandages, no instruments, save a simple wooden flute with a familiar yet strange appearance and sound. The look in his face informed me of the uneasiness he now had of bridging our simple methods to his people.

"Oh, this flute," I said, "is bait. It is just a way for me to make friends so that I can use other ways to help. I will explain to you the true medicine I bring, the medicine of the mind."

Once in my room, we made quick scheduling arrangements for the next day and Vijay, Basker, and Mitta went their way, leaving Dhamu and me alone to talk. I thought long at how I would approach the subject of hypnotism. On the table was the package brought from the stonecutters shop. A few pieces of string that had been cut from the package lay on the table beside it. I picked up a piece of string and asked Dhamu to hold his two fingers up and together. I wrapped the string around the fingers and held the ends tightly.

"Try to separate them," I said. He could not. He tugged against the string, but I applied an equal pressure, keeping his fingers bound. I unwrapped the string from his fingers and said "now imagine the string is still there holding your fingers together and try to pull them apart." I saw the little muscles in the base of the fingers flex, a familiar sign of effort, but the fingers remained together. His eyebrows rose with a look of surprise. We looked at each other then back at his fingers with wonder, then laughter. "What we think is true," I said "becomes true. Now let those fingers relax down to your side."

His arm drifted down and relaxed by his side; his hand unfolded, his eyes still transfixed on the now relaxed fingers. He looked up at me, grinned and nodded. "Programming language," He said.

"Ah, yes, Programming language."

"Now I think I understand this medicine you are bringing. Tell me, Uncle, can it help me get rid of this headache and great feeling of tiredness."

"Of course," I said, "your mind can help you with many medicines for many needs. Sit back." He sat back in the chair. "Now close your eyes and focus on your breathing. Each time you exhale, let yourself relax a little bit more." I continued guiding him through progressive relaxation of each region of the body from the toes to the head. Along the way, I gave him suggestions for release of tension and pain, along with strengthening and empowering visualizations.

He opened his eyes with a smile. "Thank you," he said. "My pain is gone, my head is clear and I feel strong in my whole body. I understand this treatment now. I think we can help many people who have been tsunami-affected in this way."

In the distance, we heard a beating drum and voices singing. "It is a funeral," he said. "They will sing like this all through the night to keep the evil away." After informing me more of the rites of the funeral, he looked at me with a far-away and curious glint in his eyes. "I want to tell you something about myself. I have done some special performances, dances with fire. People have been very happy from this performance also. It is a very exciting kind of performance, dancing around, moving the fire around me, even touching it to my body at times."

With great delight I watched his pantomime, listened to the details of his act, enjoined his widening eyes, as he recounted the tricks. With even greater widening eyes, I entered the dialogue. "Dhamu, this is a most remarkable thing. I am a fire performer. I have swallowed and blown fire while dancing, and tossed fire torches like a juggler." Our fellowship of flame was recognized without comment.

Very few can know the thrill of the flame in the rhythm and swirl of an excited audience. It is an inexplicable feeling, for fire has its own life, and unlike children or animals, it joins the performer, entices and intoxicates him. It is primal; the skillful fire performer can become as the flame itself, absorbed in glow and warmth, a force of combustion. The audience, too, experiences this first mystery, deity, awakening and engagement. If the music and mood is right, the fervor of the fire dance is divinely rapturous. With a sigh, we both exclaimed our joy at knowing this shared splendor.

"Uncle, I would like for you to tell me something. Do you think that leaders are born or made?"

"I think they must be both," I responded. "They must have certain qualities within them from birth, but they will only become leaders when the circumstance calls on them to do so and they make such a choice. None of us, Dhamu, will truly know ourselves until we have faced challenge and opportunity and seen how we will respond."

"Yes, Uncle, this is the answer I hoped I would hear. Now this is the time of deciding, of taking action, of knowing what is in us to become the leaders we were born to be. There is so much I want for my village. I want the people to have more, to have hope that their lives could be better. I know that this can only come through the education of the children so that they can improve their situation. Now, Uncle, the situation is very critical, was even critical before the tsunami came, but now is so much more difficult. I want to help the children of my village to get better education, to get a better life. That is why I worked to get the uniforms for them. That is why I thought it so important that they be able to go to their schools, properly dressed, so that they could be proud and put their attention to their studies. I hope that I have done a good thing for these children, Uncle. Do you think so?"

"Yes, Dhamu," I said, "I think you have done a very good thing for them, and I think it will make a difference in their lives for all of their time."

"Thank you Uncle, I have tried to do good." With that Dhamu left for the night. I sat at the desk and produced the small journal I had purchased at the airport in Tokyo and began to record the dream, the day, the adventure.

By now, I had developed a routine to keep the mosquitoes off me during the night. I lathered myself up with my Deet lotion and set the ceiling fan on low, crawled into bed, pulled the covers tightly around my neck, and drifted into the darkness.

I awoke rested, ready for another day. Outside the door was the morning paper. I had my breakfast snack as I read the paper and later joined Mitta at the restaurant in the hotel for a traditional Tamil breakfast of small steamed rice dumplings called "idli", a "dhosa" crepe, and ladles of a thin spicy soup, "sambar". With that my nutrition for an outing was set.

Dhamodharan met us at the hotel on his two-wheeler and Vijay was with him to help with our transport. We went to a photo shop to get pictures transferred from my camera. As we pulled up to the shop, an auto driver approached us, keenly eyeing our foreign appearance.

"Let me take you on a tour of Chennai." He solicited. "I will show you all the best sites, and I will take you to see the tsunami-affected areas also."

"I have seen them already." I said. "No thank you." But I was reminded of that long ago day as Lenise sat in the impromptu chapel in a parking lot near the recently-bombed Murrah Federal Building site in Oklahoma City. As she was giving quiet reverence to the loss of innocent lives, a woman tapped her on the shoulder. "Excuse me," she said, "can you tell me where I can buy a t-shirt?" Sadly, this tsunami tragedy had also become an attraction, and the bone-pickers had staked their turf.

Dhamodharan approached me. "Look Uncle." He pointed to a billboard across the street. On a bright yellow field, a brawny, bulky bodybuilder in an 'Incredible Hulk' flex struck a bold image. "That's it," Dhamu said. "That's my strongbody." He pointed to his head, then to his chest, then puffed up like the billboard. He seemed not only to understood, but also to embrace our strange medicine.

9

First Treatment

"Uncle," Dhamodaran said.

"Yes, Dhamu," I responded.

"Can your First Medicines help a person who has AIDS?"

"Yes, Dhamodharan, in many ways. What are you speaking of exactly?"

"I have a friend who has AIDS. He has done very well, but lately he has been very angry. I have heard him many times raising his voice with anger toward his children. I have become very concerned about him. I felt so relaxed after your treatment last night and I thought that maybe this treatment might help him. I have spoken with him already and have made arrangements to see him if you think you can help."

"Well, I think so. We will have to see."

We stopped at the internet café "browsing center" to check email messages, particularly to connect with Lenise for the first time since calling her from the airport in Singapore. The Browsing Center was a small room at the top of a flight of stairs rising from a small blacktop carport. Inside the cramped room were two rows of computer stalls, old PC's with just enough juice to chug along the information super highway or play some simple games with which the local boys seemed to be obsessed. I sent a quick note. Then, we four, Mitta riding the two-wheeler with Vijay and I aboard with Dhamu, set out for Srinivasapuram.

We zipped through the now familiar Mylapore streets, then down toward the beach, rolling slowly along the main Srini roadway. We climbed from the bikes into a crowd of children all eager to meet the foreigners, exchanged names and salutes, then walked down the narrow pathway toward Dhamu's former home. Along the pathway was a small thatched hut. We approached the entrance, but hesitated as Dhamu announced our arrival to the occupants within.

We were welcomed in like family after a long journey. A tall, lean, and drawn fellow who was approximately my own age greeted us and introduced us to his wife and two children. He offered coffee, tea, or cold drink. We sat together on plastic mats that were placed on the ground. With Dhamodharan interpreting, we asked him what was troubling him.

He told us that he was having trouble with the medicines he was taking to manage his HIV infection; they were causing his eyes and ears to itch. I asked if he had discussed this with his doctor. He replied that they told him he was having an allergic reaction and gave him some eye drops to ease the discomfort. He said that he was hesitant to use the drops because they had become filled with bubbles while he was traveling to work.

Mitta inspected the bottle of drops and assured him that the bubbles were merely from the shaking, and would settle out of the solution after a little time. I showed him a simple method to tap the bottle and release the bubbles more quickly. He was delighted with the method and smiled gratefully.

He told us that he was concerned about his temper, for he had noticed that at times he would suddenly become very angry. I asked about his sleep patterns and he said that he was not sleeping well, but had been given medicine to help him with that. I knew a certain HIV medication that was known to cause such side effects, but when we looked at his medications, it was not a part of his regimen.

He noted that he felt like a cup of tea at its fullest, ready to overflow. I responded by explaining the simple stress management strategy to empty the cup each day through relaxation and meditation in order to handle the "filling up of the cup". He was also thankful for this idea, and agreed that if he would find the time to do this each day, he could more easily keep himself from his tirades. He looked at us and asked if we could answer one more question for him. He looked at his children and then his wife, and then back to us with open eyes. "Is it possible for me to give this to my family?" Though his lips stopped moving, his eyes continued asking.

"Have they been tested?" I asked.

He replied that they had been tested and were not infected. I informed him that it was next to impossible for them to become infected unless they were to be exposed in a certain way to his blood. I explained that the virus was in his blood so he would have to be careful if he cut himself, and he should use protection when with his wife. She grinned shyly and they both affirmed that this was not an issue of concern.

Dhamodharan kept talking beyond his translation of my comments, then turned to me and said "Uncle, I have told him that his wife is his first treatment, and he should accept and enjoy her support always."

I added, "yes, and you should hold your children very close to you and let them hold you back."

His face became transformed. His eyes burst with the sorrow that had been held back for so long and streamed long tears down his face. He smiled and reached for me.

"This is the very best of news. This is what has been troubling me so and driving me to madness. This is what has been my great fear. You have given great help to me. I feel my happiness now as I have in previous times."

I offered to give him a treatment, in order to help him find his calming "empty cup" and to show his wife how she could give this very same treatment to him when he was restless. He pulled out a cloth sling-like chair that he could lay in comfortably, and we placed a small footrest under his feet so he could almost fully recline. I stepped to the head of the chair and told him to close his eyes and allow his body to relax, that each breath could allow him to relax more. I told him that I would place my hands on his head, shoulders, and other parts of his body that would also help him to relax. He instantly yielded and sank into a deep, more restive posture in the chair as I lowered my hands to rest upon his forehead and eyes.

To my astonishment, Dhamodharan began to direct him through a progressive relaxation, just as I had directed him the night before. "Now let your mind be free." I whispered and Dhamodharan echoed. "Let yourself drift to pleasant memories and dreams."

The silence was broken by a low resonant tone, a humming-like "aum" chant rising from my chest and echoing from my mouth and nose. Within moments, he picked up the tone and I felt his body vibrating in response, as I moved my hands to rest upon his shoulders.

I moved to his side, picked up his hand in mine, and holding my palm toward his, generated a field of energy that pressed against his palm. I gently placed his hand over his heart, then took his other hand and placed it over his solar plexus, resting my hands upon his. We both settled back into the song as a smile rose upon his lips, then stretched his mouth wide. He began to speak, not to me, but as though speaking in a dream.

"Tell me what you are experiencing," I said.

"I am with my family," he said, "I am feeling so happy."

His wife looked on, as if to project herself into my position in order to study the treatment method. "Enjoy yourself," I said "Let this feeling be your medicine." Then I placed her hands where mine had been.

I leaned back and produced my flute from its small bag and began to play. A canopy of profound bliss drifted down upon the room as the children gathered near, taking in the treatment scene, becoming a part of the healing soup. He told me that the music was making him feel as though he was traveling with his family and that this was making him feel strong in his whole body.

I told him to absorb this strong feeling, and to feel it renewed each day as he dressed himself. We stepped away from him and told him to be present back in the room and open his eyes when he was ready. After a few moments, his eyes opened and glistened with the same joy that had been expressed in his face.

His wife and children gathered near to him in a great family hug. Soon we all joined in with congratulatory embraces. As we all stood, he called his children before us, and thanking us, asked his children to give us a blessing. The children stepped before Mitta and me, bent forward, kissed their hands, and touched our feet. I was humbled by their expression, but accepted their gratitude with delight.

10

The Great Wave

We exited the tiny hut and stepped back into the mid-afternoon sunlight, our eyes and minds taking a few moments to adjust to the bright and busy environment. We returned to the main road and began walking toward the far end of the village, this time joined by Dhamu's friend, who walked with a renewed sense of strength. Along the road, many small children came out to greet us, introducing themselves to us, delighted to be able to use their English-speaking skills. Women sat in small groups near their homes, smiling and waving as we passed. Eventually, we came to the end of the road and walked beyond onto the sandy beach. As we walked along the beach, Dhamodharan pointed to a grassy area adjacent to the sand. On it stood a volleyball net, silent and alone.

"Here was a cricket field," Dhamu said. "On the morning of the 26th, many children, maybe forty or fifty, had gathered here to play cricket, since it was Sunday. When the wave came, it took them all away, lost to the sea."

We stood in silent awe, gazing at the empty field, imagining the sounds of the children at play, now realizing just how devastating the event was for this community.

"Here." Dhamodaran pointed to a wall of massive boulders, aligned and piled to create a levy some four feet tall, each weighing about a ton. Where he pointed along the wall was a breach, several of the stones missing from their evident positions. He pointed further inland, about

100-plus yards. "Here is where these stones were carried by the waves." We passed through the breach and toward the displaced stones. Only now did the true power of the tsunami come to me, as I saw those massive stones, about eight feet in circumference, strewn inwardly like cast dominoes. I knew the force that would be required to move the stones, and the water seemed to carry them without effort. A great hollowness grew within as we walked back toward the village.

We continued to meet many more of the villagers, especially the young fishermen who walked along the water's edge, seeming to carry desire and dread to return to the sea. We came upon a family group under a large tarp suspended by poles on the spot that had been their home. A makeshift kitchen and 'living' area were evident. The group of about seven smiled and waved as we passed then came out to greet us. A small boy stepped forward and Dhamu said, "Here is one of the village children that we have provided a school uniform for." He shook our hands and offered gratitude, which we accepted on behalf of those who had contributed. We took a photo with Dhamu and his young beneficiary and walked on. Several young boys around us were flying kites, what seemed like homemade crafts from scavenged materials.

An older gentleman approached us with a greeting. Dhamodharan informed us that his grandchild had been one of the children lost to the sea during the tsunami. We offered condolences. He informed Dhamu that his wife was still very affected by this loss. Dhamodharan offered our help and our parade turned back toward the village houses to continue the work.

We entered the small block house through a tiny patio, clouds of flies scattering as we passed. We removed our shoes and stepped one at a time into the shrinking room. They showed us the watermarks on the wall as we sat down to learn how the rising water had affected their lives. The gentleman's wife recounted how their tiny grandchild, about two years old, had been lost to the tsunami. Her sorrow flowed from every pore; her mask of profound loss was punctuated by strained, reaching, grasping, yet empty hands. She told us that this sadness had fallen heavily upon her whole family, and that she had been paralyzed by it, unable to eat or sleep, only ache in her heart. She spoke also of other pains in her body, particularly her left arm, which was swollen at the elbow from a fall she had experienced during the flight from the wave. She showed us the medicines she had been taking for her heart condition.

We sat without comment, only our attending presence. A younger woman, her friend, began to tell us of the way she was similarly suffering. She told us that her twelve-year-old daughter had been on the cricket field when the wave came and took her. She woefully reported that everything else was taken from her home by the waves, even the sewing machine from which they made their living. Her suffering was worsened because she had taken loans to pay for her daughter's education. Now she would still have to pay the loans, but with the loss of any benefit.

I remember looking at her for a long time, feeling the hopelessness, the loss compounded over and over. I could say nothing when she finished speaking, nor could any in our company. Only tears conveyed our profound sympathy. Finally, I found some words to speak.

"I am so very sorry that you are suffering in this way. It is tragic and sad that you have lost your child. In time, I hope this sadness will be softened by all the wonderful memories you have of her. There are ways that we can help you with your suffering. We can give you treatment that will help you to pass through this difficult time with less distress."

Both women agreed to receive treatments from Mitta. We moved from the tiny sitting room to an even smaller kitchen room that had only a small food prep area, storage in one corner, and what seemed like an old school bus seat. The elder woman reclined on the bench as Mitta sat to her side. Dhamu sat on the other side of the woman and Mitta began her treatment by gently touching her fingertips to several points on the woman's upper chest, near her collarbone. She then instructed the woman on how to press these same points to help resolve her distress. She placed the woman's hands by her sides, taking great care for the swollen elbow. She gently touched the arm in a sort of benediction manner, as if to anoint it and invite some healing virtue from within. She reached down, took her hand, and began to massage it gently. Keeping one hand on the woman's arm, she touched the top of her head with the other, helping her to relax her head backward as she asked her to close her eyes and begin allowing her body and mind to relax. Dhamu conveyed her instructions with passion, adding his own caring inflection to each word. Soon the woman's body yielded; she slumped into the chair and became much more at ease. I lifted my flute and began to play an accompaniment to this healing concert.

After about fifteen minutes of guided deep relaxation, with visualizations of releasing distress and becoming stronger, the woman was directed to open her eyes. The low light made her gleaming face barely visible, though somehow illumined. She reported feeling much more at ease and the arm was not hurting at all. We all celebrated her transformation toward well-being.

We invited the other woman to take her place on the bench. As she lay down on the bench, her eyes still seemed to dart about, somewhat timid and weak. Her face remained drawn downward, not quite a frown, but the congealed hollowness of deep sadness. Dhamu knew exactly what to do. With his soothing tone he began to encourage her to "let go, let go, let go." Mitta first massaged her hands, placed hands upon her head, then shoulders in a standard healing manner. She lifted the woman's hand and placed it upon her heart, holding her own hand over it as she encouraged her to be comforted in her sorrow. She told her to continue to breathe in strength and breathe out her sadness. Tears flowed from the woman's eyes, and our own. I played on, a dirge at first, but becoming hope-filled as the treatment continued. Though we all held our positions within the room, it became as though the salve of peacefulness and release bound us together as if in an embrace. Mitta gently whispered for her to take her time, and when she was ready, to open her eyes.

We waited in the silence as she absorbed her own strength. When she opened her eyes, they glistened, though not from the tears, but a sparkle that had not been present before. It was as if candles had been repositioned within the windows of her soul. These shining eyes were punctuated by a beaming smile. She looked about at all of us with a spirit of gratitude, like one who has emerged from a deep pit. She sat up on the bench and thanked us verbally, then told us she thought she would be much better now, that she must return to the needs of her family and herself, living despite the loss of her treasured daughter.

The group who had shared such despair together wallowed in the bliss of shared triumph. We spoke with them of ways we might be able to help with their other needs, particularly the possibility of purchasing rice, so they would have the physical resources to fuel their continued recovery.

We exited the tiny house into the creeping darkness of night. We walked back down the road, boarded the two-wheelers, and set out for dinner at Dhamu's family's place in town. We journeyed away from the seaside village and back into the congested city, the district of Mylapore. The roadways constantly transitioned from asphalt to dirt, turning this way and that, like a great maze. Down what seemed like an alleyway, we turned and parked. We trekked along a walkway and entered the humble but comfortable apartment to great greetings from the many family members.

Dhamu's sisters served us delicious home-cooked foods and when we were done, we spent time telling family stories, particularly enjoying the tales Dhamu's father, Narayanan, told of his youthful meeting with Jim Rudolph in the 1970's. He told how they had met one day on the beach near Srinivasapuram when Jim had strolled down the beach away from the Theosophical Society in nearby Adyar. He told how while Jim was lying in a boat reading a book, he had slinked up on him and invisibly rocked the boat in the sand, giving Jim a quick start. He told how they had embarked on a journey all around India for months. He told how they had become lifelong friends whose love was now spanning generations. He told how they had formed and sustained this relationship despite the fact that they did not speak a common language. "They communicated," Dhamu said, "through the language of brotherhood."

11

Celebrate!

As it was Vijay's birthday, we had made arrangements to join him and his family for a celebration. We zigzagged back through the Mylapore labyrinthine roads to the main road to Srinivasipuram, stopping at a small bake shop to pick up a cake. We arrived at the apartment Vijay's family was sharing with another family, due to the destruction of their own home on the beach. With great fanfare we ascended the stairs and grinned and bowed through the customary introductions. Vijay's smile beamed even brighter with the arrival at his home of his new American friends and their peculiar birthday traditions. We had no candles to place upon the cake, but we unveiled it with a rousing rendition of the birthday song, something equally foreign and entertaining.

The furnishings in the small apartment were sparse, only a couple of plastic chairs and a small television in the front room, with a large bundle of fishing nets lying beside it. Vijay stepped across the room, picked up two small items from a shelf and walked to Mitta and me. To Mitta he gave a small glass earth globe and to me a small ornate plastic dome with a decorated glass Ganesha statue within. "These are some of the few things we were able to retrieve from the rubble of our home," Dhamu translated. "They are my gift to you."

We accepted the small treasures with gratitude and reverence, marveling at the way they had been recovered and restored. We spent about an hour together, eating cake and singing the birthday song again and again. There remained a sense of somberness in our celebrations, however, for we were not the only guests in this home. Despite the delight of the birthday celebration, an undercurrent of sadness, of disruption, of alienation at being without a home, a guest in the home of another, pervaded our time together.

When we were finished with our rousing visit, we descended the stairs, climbed back upon our two-wheelers, and rocketed back to the hotel. We gathered in my room for a few last minutes together, still relishing our successful day filled with treatments, dinner, and birthday tributes. As we were saying our last goodbyes for the evening, I reached down to touch Vijay's feet in an effort to give him the same honors that I had received from the children earlier in the day. I kissed my hands and as I reached down, Vijay's feet scuttled quickly backward, like crawdads that affect a rapid retreat when confronted in the water.

"No Uncle, you must not do this!" Dhamu's reprimanding voice blurted out beside me. I stood up and looked puzzlingly at both Dhamodharan and Vijay. "It is not right; you are too much higher than Vijay for you to show such a sign of respect and devotion."

"But Vijay is to me as a brother, I do not see myself above him. On his birthday, I see him as the king and would like to give him the same blessing I have received today."

"This is our way, Uncle."

With those words I surrendered. It was not my place to defy the customs of my hosts. I felt at once insulted and ashamed. My intentions were pure and rooted in respect. A simple smile, embrace, and happy birthday would be my tribute. I also offered a gift of money, that Vijay may acquire some need or delight.

We met early the next day, our fourth in India, to run some errands. We were happy to have some open time to acquire a few materials we needed for our comfort, including some method to make tea in the room. Vijay carried a troubled look on his face. When we prodded, he told us that he had a restless night. He informed us that it was a bad omen to give him money on his birthday, that according to tradition, if he received money from another to start this year, he would become dependent on money from others to complete the year.

This tradition, of course, completely contradicted the American custom and my lifelong pleasure of birthday card cash. His logic, however, was well-reasoned. Again, it was not my place to establish new traditions, but to honor and learn from those already in place. With some sadness, I accepted the bills back from Vijay and proceeded to a nearby food counter to acquire a treat that we could all share. Our celebration, now enriched by greater understanding of each other, drifted on.

12

Project

We had made our commitment to provide school slates for the children of Muttukadu, and Dhamu said he knew just the place to acquire them. After completing our own shopping, we stopped by the Browsing Center to send an email requesting funds from Jim Uncle to purchase rice for the families we had given care. Dhamu then led us to a small shop around the corner that was more like a stall or closet than store. The counter opened directly onto the street and the clerks, two young women and a young man, rummaged through the congested space for the items we requested. After much searching and climbing, the young lad approached the counter with an armload of small school slates. We counted out thirty slates and began to negotiate our purchase.

As we were considering the importance of the slates for the children's education, it dawned on me that childhood is for more than just learning. Since the shop was packed with all manner of treasures, I turned to Dhamu and expressed my brainstorm. "Maybe they have tops, also. Children need to play as much as they need to study."

"Yes, Uncle, this is a good idea. They will have tops, and the boys will be happy with these as toys, but the girls will also need something for their delight. I would suggest jump ropes. I think it would also be a good thing to get some charts for the teachers to teach their lessons."

After some limited instruction, the clerks went searching again, and after some brief effort, emerged with an equal number of spinning tops and jump ropes. One young woman stepped forward with a roll of multi-colored language charts. With bags in arms, we mounted the two-wheelers and journeyed back to the hotel.

We had scheduled a planning session for Dhamu's project idea to visit other villages further south. Mitta, Dhamu, Vijay, and I were met by Basker and two other friends who knew the area we were interested in visiting. In my room we gathered around the bed, on which we laid out a large map of Tamil Nadu. Each of the team members had family in several villages along the coast. The plan was to go to the villages and speak with family members to find those who were tsunami-affected and offer them help. We hoped to reach Nagapattinam, the most seriously tsunami-impacted area. Dhamu had arranged for a vehicle for the week and we carefully calculated the time and costs necessary to complete the mission.

When the team had left my room, I counted out the cash I had and realized that we did not have the funds necessary to realize the project. If we were to complete Dhamu's vision to help others, we would need to acquire more money. By morning, I had a plan.

Mitta and I met Dhamu early and sat to discuss our plan. We had brought a cash stipend to pay Dhamu to help us for the three-week duration of our trip. I had paid him for his first week and had his cash payment for the remainder of his time. I had decided to send an email plea for financial support back to the US, describing the nature of our project and expected costs. I knew that the support would come, but it was unlikely to arrive before we embarked on our trip.

"Dhamu," I said, "Mitta and I have come far to help those who have been tsunami-affected in the ways that we can. We have come as volunteers, with no salaries and even paying much of our own expenses. We are not benefiting financially from our time here. If so, we would each gladly contribute more of our salaries to make this trip. I am going to need to ask you to make an investment in the project. I can apply this money to our trip budget and move forward with our plan and pay you later upon the arrival of our sponsorship funds from America."

"Uncle, you have been very helpful to my people already, and my family has benefited from my work with you. I am happy to wait for the monies until our return. Please use what you have to take this help to others." With those words, Dhamodharan went from liaison, coordinator, and aide to partner. Indeed, we had just come to help; it was his project all along.

We departed the room with a sense of resolution and purpose. Vijay waited for us with his two-wheeler at the ready. I climbed aboard with Vijay; Dhamu and Mitta boarded his two-wheeler, and the four of us set out to purchase rice.

When thinking we would buy rice, I simply thought of going to the market and purchasing several bags, but Dhamu had determined, based on Jim Uncle's email reply, that we could purchase a number of 50 pound bags. For this, we would not go to just any market, but to the rice market. We rolled down the highway past Srinivasapuram and Adyar, as though we would leave the Chennai area again, before finally arriving at a metal building, The Sakthi Wholesale Rice Merchant. It was unobtrusively set at the street with a small truck parked in front, piled high with large white bags of rice. Two men were hefting the large rice bags from the truck onto their shoulders and carrying them through a narrow doorway, sweating from their burdens in the hot sun.

We dismounted from the bikes and, after stretching a bit to release stiffened muscles, passed through the door into the warehouse. Before us stood a group of men gathered around a large table. On the table lay over one hundred small trays filled with a vast array of different types of rice: short, long, brown, white, etc. The rice dealers sat at one end of the table as buyers strolled along the table lifting the trays, pinching, dropping, inspecting the different varieties and grades. The room was piled high with columns of rice bags and at the far end of the small room, a doorway opened into a maze-like warehouse filled with stack after stack of the large bags.

"Dhamodharan, I had no idea there were this many different types of rice."

"Yes Uncle, this is why we have come here. We can get the best rice for our people at the best price."

Soon, our turn at the table arrived and we stepped to the table mimicking the gestures of the previous buyers, lifting this grain then that grain, trying to take in the seemingly infinite considerations. Dhamodharan began his dealings with a man at the end of the table who soon disappeared and returned with yet another variety. Dhamodharan inspected it, turned to me and stated "Uncle, this is the rice we need." Then Dhamu began an energetic, if not heated, negotiation over price. In time the discussion, though still intense, had both men nodding in agreement. "Uncle, we have been given a good price, and they have agreed to deliver it to the village also." Another man emerged and began writing the invoice, which Dhamodharan paid with the money sent by Jim.

Satisfied, we exited the warehouse, climbed aboard the two-wheelers, and jaunted back to Srinivasapuram.

Upon arriving in the village, we went directly to Dhamu's friend to determine his outcome from our treatment. Finding no one at home, we strolled back down the main roadway to visit with the women we had also treated. Again, the knocks at the door were unanswered. We turned back to go to Vijay's and await the delivery of the rice.

13

First Clinic

We walked down the village roadway as sweet, celebratory music spilled out from a small inner "street", giving us a sense of rhythm and sway to our stroll.

"Uncle, there is a wedding taking place. For someone, this is their special happy day."

We walked on, waving to the villagers at their business or sitting in their clusters. As we passed one house, a gentleman about my age stood and greeted us. Noticing the camera dangling about my neck, he said "Photo" and struck a stoic pose. A much older white-haired man stood beside him in a similar manner. I turned to take their photo then negotiated my way over a watery mud hole to show them the image on my display, a great boon in the age of digital cameras. He was excited to see himself and his friend looking so handsome and impressive in the photo. Two women, one older, the other perhaps her daughter, stepped up to our gathering beside the autorickshaw and took their turn at being photographed. We all shared a delightful exchange over the photos, each happy for their own novel experience.

The younger man turned to Dhamu and asked why we were in the village. Dhamu informed him that we had come to offer help to those who were "tsunami-affected" and we were there today to follow up on treatments we had given. At this news, the man gently recoiled with a twisting movement and looked at me with a sense of pleading as he reached to demonstrate the discomfort he was carrying in his neck and shoulders. He told Dhamu that he had been in bad pain for some time, as though it was, clenching his fists and shaking his arms, within his very bones. He had also been dizzy and very fatigued.

Noting his report and his now-revealed mask of pain, I told Dhamu that we would be happy to offer him a treatment. At this the older of the women complained that she had been experiencing terrible neck and head pain also. Standing still beside the fly-gathering muck, I began to look about for an appropriate place to sit for a treatment. The woman led us to a door across the alleyway and opened it to reveal a hidden courtyard. Stepping into the courtyard, I proclaimed "this will do nicely."

Two plastic chairs were brought in and set side by side as the now-growing company flowed into the courtyard behind us. The gentleman sat in one chair and the woman in the other, with Mitta standing beside her. I had been taught a Chinese pulse diagnosis method to identify pain in the body, so I decided to check the gentleman's pulse to see if I could assess the manner of his pain. As I reached to place my hand upon his wrist, I instantly noted an intense rigidity in his entire arm. I lifted the arm at the wrist and the entire arm moved like that of a plastic action figure. I lifted the other arm and found the same condition. If I was going to help this fellow with his pain through hypnotic relaxation, I thought, I was going to have to get a good start by getting these arms to relax.

I reached down and took hold of his right thumb and instructed him, through Dhamu's assistance, to let his arm just dangle as I lifted it. This method is used to allow and assess the release of control of the arm. It is commonly used after hypnotic induction as a deepening technique, but I knew I would need to start here in order to initiate the first stages of relaxation. In practice, the whole arm is dangled by the thumb and then released to fall to the side. The drop and effect of the weight serves to deepen the level of relaxation. If, upon release, the arm does not drop, it is an indication that the individual is still 'holding on', which will inhibit their overall depth response. In this gentleman's case, I lifted and swayed the arm, yet its rigidity caused his whole body to move. As I released the arm, it continued to hang in the air like a stone sculpture. I lifted the other arm and found the same response. I repeated the action again and again, eventually taking both thumbs at the same time, wiggling, and thrusting the arms downward to his thighs. After several repetitions, he finally yielded; his shoulders relaxed and he slumped in the chair.

His eyes were already closed as I stepped behind the chair, placing one hand on his shoulder and the other atop his head. Dhamu guided him to be mindful of his breathing, to release tension with each exhalation, and to feel his muscles relaxing and becoming more and more comfortable from head to toe. I reached around his head and placed my hand on the center of his chest. His head rolled gently backward to rest upon my upper torso as he let out a sigh and sank deep into bliss, punctuated with a bright yet passive smile. With his gentle and encouraging voice, Dhamodharan continued to almost whisper in his ear then turned to me. "I have sent him to get his strongbody, Uncle."

Beside us, Mitta had begun to give care to the woman simply by massaging her shoulders and neck. Dhamodharan turned to help with guided instructions. He guided her through breathing release and head to toe relaxation. Mitta moved from working on her shoulders to massaging hands, then feet. Dhamu checked with the woman to see how she was feeling and learned that her pain had dissipated and she was feeling much better.

He returned to where I had been working with the gentleman. I had moved from his head and chest to holding his hands, one and then the other, between my two palms, then giving the same treatment to his lower legs. Vijay and Basker stood nearby, studying every movement and gesture, stepping in to assist by placing their own hands where mine had been. Afterward, the man reported that his pain had gone away, that he was feeling much better, and more confident. We informed him that his body now knew what to do to give him comfort. We awakened him from his hypnotic slumber and encouraged him to seek medical attention for his condition.

The older man had taken his place upon a plastic mat that was brought into the courtyard and placed before the chairs. I turned my attention toward his care with Dhamu there to translate and lend his now-developing therapeutic manner. A group had continued to gather in the courtyard, and now two other villagers took their turns in the chairs. The music from the wedding continued to drift through the village, swirling about in the courtyard to give us a cadence by which to work. Our improvised clinic became a pageant of care as villager after villager took their place in the chairs to share their aches and sorrows and receive our special treatments.

Now the young woman, whom we had first met on the street, also stepped in to help with the treatments. To my astonishment, I watched her lift and drop the hands of the villagers as she had seen me do earlier. Dhamu, Vijay, and Basker similarly "prepped" the villagers for treatment, now understanding the guided relaxation and release process and simply relying on Mitta and me to hear the specifics of their complaints and give direct visualization or manipulation guidance.

Most of the villagers receiving treatment presented complaints unrelated to the tsunami. One gentleman, the resident of the home we had commandeered, complained of long-term pain and swelling in a leg that had been injured in a fight. He led me into his small home and I instructed him on how to elevate his leg to help with the swelling as I guided him through hypnotic pain relief. After his treatment he brought his son, a lad of about ten who wore a cast on his right arm. His arm had been broken when he was captured and tumbled by the tsunami. The boy complained that the arm was "itchy". I informed him that the itchiness was a sign that his arm was healing. I seated him in the chair and asked him to close his eyes and see himself playing with his friends.

"I am playing cricket with my friends." He said.

"That's good," I replied. "Every day close your eyes and imagine yourself playing this game. Think of the time that your arm will be completely healed, your cast will be removed, and you will return to play with your friends. You will find that time comes very soon." He rose from the chair and thanked us, reporting that his arm now felt comfortable and strong.

The searing midday sun settled behind the adjacent building. The music continued as day turned to evening and then night. As we were concluding our clinic, a young woman approached holding a young child. She informed us that she had been very distressed since her flight from the tsunami with her children, fearful that they would all be lost.

Mitta approached her. "Sit here and let one of the others hold your child for a few moments," Dhamu translated. "Tell me what is troubling your heart. Close your eyes and tell me what you see."

"I am running." The woman stated. We are all so scared. The wave is behind us and we are afraid it will swallow us. I have my children with me and I am carrying my baby. We do not know what will happen. I don't want to die. I don't want my children to die. I see a bird, a parrot that is flying overhead. He is flying above us, he is safe."

"Think of this parrot." Mitta said. "Feel his safety within yourself. You are safe now. You have survived tsunami. This parrot is now telling you to remember. You are safe now. Think of this parrot often and each time, remember that you are safe."

She opened her eyes, reached out and embraced Mitta, then gathered her baby and children to return to her home.

We exchanged many embraces and hands-clasped bows of "Vanakam Nanthree" with the villagers who were lingering in the courtyard. We were exhilarated. I lost track of how many people we treated. Our vigor superseded our fatigue, so we sat and rested while reviewing the many remarkable moments we had observed throughout the afternoon. The music from the nearby wedding continued to play, a soundtrack to our fulfilling day.

During our clinic, word came that the rice truck had arrived, and Vijay went to his home to help unload and place the bags in a storage area. We gathered our things and walked the block or so to Vijay's. We first delivered a bag to Dhamu's friend whom we had treated the day before. His family greeted us with cheers and embraces. He informed us that he was feeling great since his treatment, "happy, like in previous times."

The same occurred at each of the two families we had offered treatment to on the previous day. They reported their pains and sorrows had been rinsed away and received our gift of food with glee. We also delivered rice to a young woman and daughter living alone near Dhamu's old home.

Finally, we loaded a bag onto Vijay's two-wheeler and rode back to Dhamu's home in Mylapore. The rice was received with gratitude and we were rewarded with a delicious chapatti dinner. The spices, textures, and sauces tasted somehow like a medicine, a feast, ambrosia of gods.

14

Special Thali

As previously mentioned, for my protection through the night, I developed a pattern of applying mosquito spray to my face and arms, setting the ceiling fan on an appropriate speed to keep the air stirred, and securing my covers around my neck. There, I would lie motionless sleeping through the night, active in my dream workshop. In the morning, the incessant beeping of high-pitched horns on the street would stir me from my sarcophagus-like sleep sanctuary. Upon arising, I did just a bit of stretching before opening the curtains to the glorious day. After some meditation, I would gather the daily paper deposited at my door and read it while enjoying my early breakfast snack. Later, Mitta and I would have a traditional South Indian breakfast at the restaurant in the basement.

As today was the day for our project to move south, I packed my bags in preparation for departing the hotel. We had arranged for Dhamu to arrive at noon, but at 10:00 a knock came at my door. "Uncle, we are all here and ready to go. The driver is waiting downstairs with the car."

I took a few minutes to complete my packing as Vijay and Basker arrived to carry our bags to the waiting Toyota Land Cruiser with driver and new team member, Dessapan. We completed our business at the front desk and said our farewell to the MGM Grand Hotel. Our first stop was at the Browsing Center to send a report to the States. I wrote an email for Lenise to forward to our contacts, telling of the tremendous success we had the night before and our plan to take this same service to others. I included a plea for sponsorship for our efforts. Lenise learned that Western Union was waving fees for funds sent to the tsunami zone, so she would coordinate the transfer of funds from our donors in the U.S. to India.

By the time we reached the outskirts of Chennai and Adyar, it was lunchtime. Dhamu recommended that we stop at an "American Hotel". We stopped at a comfortable-looking location and walked through the open space on the first floor toward the "AC" sign that designated an air conditioned room in the basement. Our team sat at a large booth to enjoy our first meal together, celebrating the launch of our endeavor. Dhamu recommended that I try the "Special Thali Meal".

Soon, the waiter arrived with a large platter piled high with white rice, encircled with many small cups filled with all manner of sauces and relishes. Another waiter arrived with a small bucket and ladle. Dhamu nodded to the waiter and he ladled a small amount of what I would later learn was ghee or clarified butter on top of the pile of rice. Dhamu next instructed me to pile this sauce, then this relish atop the rice. I mixed the concoction together with the fingers of my right hand and surrendered myself to this culinary delight. In turn, Dhamu would instruct me to add this sauce or to sip from this bowl or that as the others looked on, enjoying their own meals, but relishing my enjoyment of the feast even more. Hot, cool, sweet, thick, and thin the sauces flowed and my palate rejoiced. The waiter came with another bucket and heaped another pile of rice upon my platter, to which the same choreographed epicurean ecstasy began anew. At the end, a single small green banana was produced, a cooling dessert. To my astonishment, the price for the feast was 42 rupees, about one dollar. The mysteries of India were indeed delectable.

Happily stuffed, we piled back into the Cruiser and set out for Muttukadu. The now familiar sites rolled past us as Tamil Super 8 film music blared from the stereo. We were excited to finally be under way. We passed the MGM Dizzy World amusement park which indicated our destination was near. Minutes later we arrived at the vast tent encampment we had visited less than a week before.

We greeted Ramalinga and Sathish, joyous at our return, and informed them we had some school supplies for the children. We were led to an open-sided tent that sported a banner for the Christian Children's Fund. Along the way, we passed the huts. Previously just frames, they were now completed with walls and roofs. Rows of hut frames stood at the ready for their own completion.

Once in the tent, the teachers greeted us and offered a seat as the children began to arrive. They were seated orderly before us, as though some program was about to take place and we were the featured presentation. The brightly-colored clothing on the preschool children reminded me of the multi-colored gumdrop and licorice allsorts candy displays I had seen at a festival in Geneva. Each child smiled their brilliant smiles, their eyes giving the greatest of gifts to all in our company.

As the time passed while the children were arriving, I realized we were all waiting for a show, so I asked if any of the children had a song that they would like to share. One girl, about age seven, instantly stood and began to sing. We all applauded, so she began the song again. After a couple of rounds of the song, another stood and sang and then another. Encouraged by the flow, the first girl stood again and recited a poem. I had carried my flute into the tent and began to play for the children, teachers, and parents who had gathered. We passed time in this way, alternating our presentations until all had gathered to fill the pavilion. One of the teachers stepped forward to tell us that the song the little girl had just sung was a song about the tsunami and how they had struggled to escape from the wave.

The teachers then opened a folder from which they produced drawings that the children had made of their flight from the wave. One particular drawing struck me; an image of all blue with wave-like lines in which were houses, boats, and trees turned this way and that with several people interspersed, captions rising from them. It truly depicted the mayhem which this child had experienced. On the back was a narrative of the event. When I said how much I liked the drawing, the teacher removed it from the folder and presented it to me as a gift. She then offered one of the drawings to Mitta. I suggested that it might be good to have the children make drawings and songs speaking of how their lives would be when they had recovered their homes again after tsunami.

Dhamu stepped forward with the charts. Together we unrolled them and presented them to the teachers. They then gathered the smaller children and began to bring them forward as the stack of slates, brought from the Cruiser by Vijay, was passed forward. Dhamu, Mitta, and I were given the honor of distributing a slate to each of the children in need. A few extras remained for those students that had not made it to the tent. The teachers received the tops and jump ropes with the promise to distribute them appropriately.

Our presentations complete, we exited the pavilion to a setting sun and a pageant of young girls at play nearby. Our procession wound through the huts and frames into the tarpaulin tent section of the camp, arriving at a clear area where mats had been placed for us to do our work. The young boy we had met before was brought to us by his mother. He still had his pouted, protruded lower lip and glassy gaze. I encouraged his mother, like his father before, to continue to embrace and reassure him. I produced my flute from my bag and began to play. I turned slightly away from the boy and played into the open air. His gaze fixed on my playing and he seemed to rest a little deeper into his mother's arm. Dhamu and the rest had now gathered around, along with several villagers.

"I play," I told Dhamodharan, "as though I am playing for this tree. In this way our friend can enjoy the music without having to directly receive and respond to it. If I were to turn and play directly toward him, it would be too much. He would recoil and become distressed." I put the flute to my lips and continued to play.

"Yes, Uncle, it seems that he has come a little out from himself to hear your song."

My song was interrupted by the arrival of the young girl with facial paralysis, Monika, and her father. There was no apparent change in her condition, but her father informed us that the doctors had recommended massage and were now treating her with electro-stimulation. We were encouraged to know our treatment was on the right track. I placed hands on Monika's face as I had before and our eyes smiled with gratitude into each other's.

When the treatment was complete, Dhamu leaned toward me. "Uncle, I am going to go for a few minutes to check on others. You will be fine here while I am gone."

I protested his departure, but he left anyway, leaving us with no way to speak to our newfound friends. I sat awkwardly for a few moments, but felt it was up to me to engage the group. A small child sat before me, so I began to entertain her with magic tricks. I began with the sliding separated finger, moved on to the appearing and disappearing fingers, and concluded with some coin tricks. Then I taught her how to do the coin stashes and productions. Who needed words when we had magic!

My list of tricks now played out and Dhamu still away, I began to think fast of some other entertaining distraction. I turned to Basker and requested a small piece of paper. From the paper I folded and tore a smaller piece, about a three-inch square. I began to fold the paper this way and that. The children and their parents leaned closer to see what was coming next. Absent my ability to provide patter during the exercise, I meticulously made and creased each of the twenty-seven folds. Finally, I folded out my fingers and palms to present a small white origami dove. Excitement and applause erupted.

I turned to Basker and requested more paper, distributing pieces to each of the group members, mostly Tamil fishermen about my age and a few children. I guided each through this fold then that. We compared our individual projects at each turn to make sure we were all on track together. There were no words, only gestures and nods of approval. I thought back to my own instruction in this craft, how twenty years earlier I had learned to fold this crane/dove from a Japanese woman, a waitress, who spoke no English. Here this skill was being passed again without the use of language, only universal communication through art.

We heard a screech and bang on the roadway about fifty yards away. Mitta and I gathered our belongings and made our way to the road to investigate. Upon arrival, we found that a motorcyclist had crashed, but the crowd around the rider had helped him gather himself and his bike from the hazard of the road. The bike was somewhat damaged with the handlebars twisted and a light broken, but the rider seemed unharmed.

In the darkness, amidst the black-skinned Tamils, I noticed another westerner. He told us he was there with a friend, a local man now living in Philadelphia, who was leading a project to provide fishing boats for this village. The local man approached us and asked what we were doing there. We informed him of our work to help those traumatized by the tsunami. When we mentioned hypnosis, he dismissingly told us that the villagers had their temple system to tend to their emotional needs and we were out of place. We tried to explain the nature of our work in greater detail as Dhamodharan arrived and engaged in an intense Tamil discourse. Soon the older man began to nod with assent. This went on for a couple of minutes and finished with what appeared to be words of salutation toward Dhamu. The man turned to us and spoke in English, "your friend is a very good propagandist for your work, and very well-spoken." With that, we were troubled no more.

As the crowd dispersed, we returned to our place in the camp where Dhamu had brought a woman who complained of having a headache on one side of her head, pain throughout her body, and trouble eating and sleeping. Mitta had her lie down on the mat and gave her a relaxation treatment while placing hands on her head and massaging her shoulders and hands. I played flute in the background as Dhamu translated Mitta's instructions. After about ten minutes of treatment, the woman reported feeling much better, that her headache had subsided. Mitta encouraged her to drink plenty of fresh water and eat food to regain her strength.

Before our departure, there was one more formal meeting for us to make. We gathered in a secluded tent, me, Dhamu, Mitta, Basker, Vijay, and Eswari his fiancée, or "would-be". Vijay and Eswari sat side-by-side before us. Vijay presented her to us. We wished happiness and blessing on both of them and all the goodness for their future marriage.

Night now fully descended, we said our goodbyes and climbed back into the Cruiser to head for Mamallapuram. We arrived at a much different location than we had previously visited, the beach hotel and tourist strip. Dhamu suggested we remain near the vehicle as he and the driver went in to negotiate a fair rate for the night. A few minutes later they returned with the good news that they had rooms for all in our company at a very good price. We loaded our baggage into our rooms then strolled down the dirt road, lined on each side by shops, to the beach. Here boats had been dragged far up on the sand. A local informed us that during the tsunami the entire area had been flooded by the waves.

It had been a long and full day. Our project was now fully underway and we had enjoyed our first successes in Muttukadu. We walked back from the beach toward the busier area of the village, our appetites leading us toward some new reward.

"Uncle," Dhamodharan said, "I am beginning to understand these first medicines more now. I can see how with such simple ways we have helped to give hope to those who are suffering from tsunami. It is as though we are lighting a fire within them to bring them back to health. I think, Uncle, that this is a flame which can light the whole world."

"Yes Dhamu, I think you truly are coming to understand these first medicines. Like me, you are beginning to feel this fire stirring inside. It seems such a simple thing and yet it is so remarkably powerful for the one who is in need."

15

Rolling

I awakened to an eerie silence. Absent were the ubiquitous sounds of city life: the clamor, the rush, and beep-beeping of everyone, at once and continually. I lay still in my bed for some time, perhaps slipping back to dreams before stirring. When I had fully awakened, I lay listening to the nothingness; in the distance, sounds of life beckoned me from my shroud. I arose, dressed, and stepped out into the Mamallapuram morning. The hotel was quiet and I walked downstairs to find the same stillness. Out on the street, the village was just awakening. The cool morning air and casual rhythm were like a living poem.

I strolled out into the street, now in the light of morning, enjoying the multicolored signs and banners that lined it. Like no other place I had been since arriving in India, this was clearly a western-flared locale, a backpacker destination. Close to the hotel I even saw a sign near an Ayurveda clinic reading "Reiki". Dr. Usui would be happy indeed to know how his "discovery" had spread throughout the world, even to this tranquil 1,300 year old tourist site. Feeling somewhat at home as in Venice Beach, I sauntered down the dusty street to take in more of its treasures. About a block from the hotel was an internet browsing center. The sign in the window stated that they opened at 10am, two hours hence. Further down the street was a music shop. I looked into the window for a flute, but seeing none, decided to return later when it opened. After some time, I returned to the hotel and found Dhamu and the guys awake and lingering near the hotel, anxious to continue the work.

Soon Mitta arrived, informing us that she had had her own excursion and found a pleasant European-styled terrace café that served a nice breakfast nearby. We set a plan to enjoy some time in the village and check in at the browsing center before continuing on. I was happy to hear about some home-styled food, so as the guys went out for their fare and Mitta went to get an Ayurvedic oil massage, I treated myself to a vegetable omelet at the terrace restaurant. I denied myself a nice espresso so as to not suffer another withdrawal. I enjoyed the quiet overlook of the strip and the beach. There was a small altar with a seated Buddha figure near one wall, seeming a bit out of place in this domain of so many Ganesha figures.

After breakfast I stopped back by the music shop. I ventured inside and inquired about flutes. It has been a long tradition to seek flutes everywhere I go. I made my first purchase of a small bamboo flute in a junk shop called The White Elephant Shop on Santa Monica Boulevard in West Hollywood in 1984. The shopkeeper was surprised that I was willing to pay five dollars for what seemed like a toy. This first flute was followed by many more, several purchased as gifts by Lenise, which have accumulated to a constantly growing collection over the decades. While in India, I thought it most appropriate to seek the signature Indian flute, the snake charmer flute, called Makudi. To my delight the shop owner produced one from behind the counter. The gourd reed flute was a bit challenging to play at first, but I soon produced a few tones, near notes, and negotiated a reasonable price. During our exchange, I was told yet another story of how the tsunami had flooded this very shop and the owner was only now returning it to operating order. My patronage became another means to aid recovery.

I returned to the hotel to show off my new flute and as I began to play it for the guys, they rushed me, saying "do not play that flute here; if you play that flute, you will cause the snakes to come." I put the flute away, but felt somehow encouraged that I had, indeed, made an authentic purchase.

By mid-morning we had completed our tasks, were loaded back into the cruiser and on our way to our next adventure. We bobbed and swayed to the Tamil music, rolling down the highway watching fields, small temples, oxcarts, and other visual treats pass us by.

In time I began to notice white mounds in marsh-like fields. I soon realized that this was salt manufacturing taking place in the simplest of ways, by hand labor. I recognized the workers raking the crystals from the lagoons and accumulating them into the small piles. The driver turned into a lot on the side of the road. Beside a field worker's hut was a glistening pile of white crystals. I was reminded of the story of Gandhi taking his walk to the sea in order to make salt and now imagined him in this place.

I was stirred from my reverie by the voice of Basker beside me. He reached out his closed hand and said "My gift to you." I placed my hand beneath his and watched as the crystals descended from his hand into mine. I clutched the salt like I would gold, marveling at is splendor and significance. I placed it in a small bag and tucked it safely into my backpack as we loaded up to move on.

Some distance further, we stopped at a small shop to "provide relief" at their facilities. Under a large tree near the road, a woman stood by a wooden table, a cluster of ripe coconuts hanging from a rope in the tree beside her. Dhamu approached her and negotiated our fair "Indian" price as we each lined up to enjoy the delicious treat. She raised a great and aged knife high and dropped it with force, opening the shell and exposing the tender treat. The milk refreshed us and as we returned to the road, the soft coconut meat provided just the sustenance to keep us moving on.

After more bobbing and rolling, we stopped at a building along the roadside. "Uncle, we will look here at boats. This is the best place to acquire them, so we will look to see what kind of boat will be best for Vijay." We walked around to the side of the building and spoke to some workers who directed us to a thatched-roof pavilion a few yards away. Inside the pavilion were several large wooden forms with fiberglass panels built inside, elements of the boats we found under construction in an adjacent pavilion. Another worker directed us through the projects underway, explaining how the strips of fiberglass cloth were layered with the resin over the forms to create the elements of the now nearly complete boats. The smell of the resins, fiberglass, and solvents were a bit overwhelming and the choking dust from their sanding made the pavilion totally inhospitable. Even though it was the only shaded refuge from the encroaching mid-day heat, we retreated into the sunshine and sprinted to the car.

Back within the comfort of air-conditioning, we continued our trek. In time we arrived at what was by now a familiar scene, a dirt road off the main highway leading past fields toward the sea. We had reached our first village destination. As we drove into the village, we noticed that things seemed somewhat orderly, unlike the mayhem in Muttukadu. Basker jumped out of the cruiser and disappeared for a few minutes to search for his relatives, returning to tell us to drive on. We continued through the village, eventually arriving at a temple, a large colorful concrete building. Next to the temple was a police station. There was a small crowd gathered before the building and several policemen stood among them. As we pulled up near the crowd, the villagers and police approached the vehicle. Dhamu instructed us to remain inside as he hopped out to exchange information. As he stood speaking with the police, several of the villagers encircled the vehicle, gazing in to observe the strange visitors. We waved our greetings to the strangers, as curious about them as they were of us.

Soon, Dhamu returned to the vehicle. "Uncle it is not good for us here. There have been some problems and we will not be able to do our work here, but there is one here who desires to speak with you."

I exited the vehicle and followed Dhamu over to a young man who stood before the temple with a few others standing near him. "Uncle he has a disease of the liver, hepatitis. He heard that you are a therapist and is wondering if there is anything you can do to help him."

I asked if he had been receiving care and he reported that he had, but he was looking for ways to help himself. I told him we were unable to provide service while there. When he reported that he had family near Srinivasapuram and would travel there to see us, we left the contact exchange for Basker, whose family could help him locate us.

On the way out of the village, Dhamu reported that there had been trouble with violence between two families that had spilled over into factions within the village. A murder had been committed about a year before and now someone had returned to the village that was re-igniting the tumult. That is why the police had been on station there, to keep the embers from stirring to flame.

We drove back down the narrow dirt road, admiring the colorful floating butterflies and darting gossamer-winged dragonflies that buzzed along the tall marshy grasses. We turned back onto the blacktop and continued our drive.

16

Village Kalapeta

We drove a few kilometers on, down the same blacktop highway, a bit set back in our aspirations, realizing that some barriers to care could not be breached. We held on to our hopes. The next stop would be different.

We turned again down a small road that led to another coastal village. The same scenes greeted us as we drove through the fields with grass-filled ditches lining the road; a farmer and his ox were working in the marshy field. We entered the Village Kalapeta, stopping at a small house. Vijay and Basker jumped out, asking us to wait for them to find family members and seek approval from the village elders for us to do our work. In time they returned to the vehicle and directed us down a smaller road. The driver parked and we disembarked. We were led past huts, down a winding trail to an open area near the beach. Palm trees formed a perfect canopy overhead, shading us from the afternoon sun.

A mat and chair were brought out for us, a now-familiar sign that our work was about to begin. A parade of villagers followed, Basker in the lead, and took seats in a circle around the area. About thirty villagers, mostly women, eventually arrived to join us. Sitting on the concrete foundation of a house no longer there, I spoke to the group. Through Dhamu's aid, I told them that we had come to offer them simple ways to help reduce their suffering, ways that if they were to watch and learn, they could use for themselves after we left. They nodded with curios anticipation.

A woman about thirty years old was brought to us, though the manner of her walk and posture made her look much older. She stepped slowly, tilted to one side, grimacing as she moved. Clearly in pain, she winced and held her side as she took a seat. She was aided by a friend who looked on with concern. The woman told us that she had been tumbled by the tsunami and carried a distance, crashing into several objects and swallowing sea water. She rasped as she breathed, her voice weak as she reported her painful ordeal. She said that she had been to the doctors and received medicine, but her condition continued to worsen.

We asked for permission to place our hands on her. She invited it and replied that it would be like being touched by a god. I told Dhamu that I was not altogether comfortable with that notion, but understood it as their way and their medicine.

Mitta began the treatment by simply massaging her hands, working on the areas of the hand known to help treat the lungs. I placed my hands on her head and then her shoulders, simply letting them rest in place as I instructed Dhamu in guided relaxation, taking time to slowly relax her and bring comfort to her body. Her friend studied our movements and methods and soon joined in on the treatment, massaging her feet and looking on with great caring eyes as her friend settled into her relief. I stepped aside as Mitta and the friend continued the treatment. I produced my flute and began to play as Dhamu continued to implore her to relax, relax, relax and let go.

From my backpack, I produced an aromatic oil blend of eucalyptus and tea tree oil, along with others to help with the lungs. Lenise had purchased the oil and used it to treat her mother through a bout of pneumonia years earlier and had sent it with me to help strengthen and protect me in this foreign environment. I took a paper napkin from my pack and soaked it with the oil. At first I held the pad near the woman's mouth and nose and asked her to slowly breathe it in. After a few moments she had the strength to take hold of the pad herself as she slowly inhaled the therapeutic fumes. Within about two minutes she stirred from her slump and began to cough. Through her coughing she was able to bring up some mucus from her lungs, which she spit upon the ground. She took hold of the chair and uprighted herself, drawing in a deeper breath.

We gave her friend another sop of the oil, wrapped in plastic to keep it from drying, and told her to let her breathe it when she wanted. We also instructed the friend to make sure she got plenty of fresh water and to take her for short walks when she could, particularly helping her to get some warming sunshine. I learned later that Mitta also gave the friend some money for more medical treatments.

Several other villagers were brought to us complaining of familiar concerns: headache, body ache, sleeplessness, and loss of appetite. Some reported that their bodies actually began to shake when they even heard the word "tsunami". We treated them all in the same manner, at times seeing actual pleas for us to place hands upon them and offer relief from this "tsunami trauma syndrome". We helped them to restore their sense of well-being, to be free from their pain, and to be reassured that they were now safe, to know they had indeed survived the tsunami and could have strength to recover and rebuild. They thanked us graciously, rising from the chair to return to their lives.

After treating villagers for about two hours, two women brought us a young boy about six years of age. He had burn scars from his face to his feet and was a little drawn and tense. He looked around with inquisitive eyes but did not speak, only smiled a little. The women told us that he had been burned when less than one year old and that a fever some time after had caused him to suffer damage to his brain.

Several of the village women gathered around, like an array of aunties, all concerned over the welfare of the child. As we laid him down upon the mat, he looked up at me with trusting eyes. I felt embraced by this group, permitted into their circle of care. He looked from me to one and then the other with the same trusting and thanking eyes. I began to gently rock his body and felt it relax and surrender to the rhythm. His arms and legs broke free from their rigidity and floated toward the ground. He became like water flowing, flowing into a calm pool. The women looked on as I instructed them in the method and one by one reached out to take hold, to give their own care through this gentle rocking touch.

I sat back from the group, picked up my flute and began to play, giving soundtrack to this symphony of compassion, observing how one in need had brought so many to this moment of fulfillment. After some time of treatment, I recommended to the mother that she give him regular massages with coconut oil to help keep the scar tissues soft and the muscles more relaxed.

We packed up our bags, rolled up the mat, and made our return parade from this oasis of care on the beach. Several of the villagers had complained of having "tsunami cough", so we prepared several blotters of the oil and distributed them. The woman who had brought her sick friend thanked us for giving her tools to provide relief and said she felt confident she could continue with these methods. We had, all of us, been through a tremendous experience of shared caring. We faced each other with hands before our chests, saying "Vanakam Nanthree" as we turned toward the vehicle.

I looked back toward this now vacant spot on the beach. We had arrived at a place that still bore the wounds of the violent waves. I saw echoed shadows of the circle of villagers who had come to receive and give care. What I saw in departure was a different place than the one at which I had arrived. Perhaps, I thought, when passing this spot in the future, these villagers would not think of the destruction and loss, but of the breezy afternoon when strangers came to comfort them and teach them ways to comfort each other.

The mood in the vehicle was transformed to one of celebratory exaltation. We reviewed the various treatments and their outcomes and spoke of our concerns for ongoing support, particularly for the woman who was still so weakened from her injuries. I remembered the method developed by Emil Coué that involved tying twenty knots in a cord and repeating an affirmation of well-being such as "every day, in every way, I am better and better." Since it was becoming clear that we needed to deliver not just care, but also tools for ongoing care, I considered that this may be a good method to teach. I had packed a ball of cotton twine, along with other supplies for disaster support, and rummaged through my bag to find and produce it. I retrieved my Swiss Army Knife from my backpack and cut a length of the cord to begin tying knots.

Vijay saw my knife and asked to examine it. I passed it to the back of the cruiser where he and Basker and Dessapan each took a turn at opening and inspecting this tool and that tool with great wonder. Clearly, they had never seen such a multi-faceted tool and demonstrated to each other how this or that blade would be used. I realized that this type of tool would be a truly grand kit for a Tamil fisherman. I then realized that as fishermen, they would have the skill to produce the knotted cords that we could use in our clinics. I passed them the ball of twine and, tying a couple of knots to demonstrate size and spacing, asked them to produce small cords of twenty knots. They took on the project with enthusiasm, soon presenting me with a short cord of twenty of the most elegant knots, equally spaced and perfectly sized.

As we conducted our rolling workshop, the road carried us to Pondicherry, where we would rest for the night. We passed through a large concrete arch and Dhamu said "Uncle, we are now in Pondicherry district, see how it is different here. This is the area of India that belonged to France and still has its style from that country."

My first observation was the difference of the police officers who wore upright red caps similar to those seen in the film *Casablanca*. We had arrived in the city at rush hour and the streets were highly congested with bicycles, another stark difference from Chennai. While many autorickshaws continued their beep-beep-beeping, the unmistakable sound of bicycle bells rang out across the boulevards. The bicyclists also seemed to navigate like schools of fish through the flowing traffic.

We stopped for an early dinner at an elegant air-conditioned American Hotel then traveled a few blocks to the Jaya Inn where we found comfortable accommodations. There was a browsing center across the street from the hotel, so I checked emails and downloaded images from my digital camera. The manager of the center was fluent in English and I learned that there was a browsing center a few blocks away that had phones from which I could call the USA.

The night had wrapped the city in darkness and the street bazaar near the hotel was packing up as Mitta joined me on my trek to the phone. I called Lenise and heard her voice for the first time in ten days. It was the longest period we had gone without speaking directly in our twenty-one years together. I told her about our good day's work, of the great outcomes we had experienced and the splendorous sights I had seen. In this strange and mysterious place, on the other side of the world, I listened to her soothing voice for a few precious minutes, feeling the comfort of family and home, a grand finish to a good day.

17

Lazarus

Kunimeddu resembled each of the other villages we had visited. First were small roads, some asphalt and some dirt, lined with small concrete block homes. The roads led to the beachfront where the block homes gave way to thatched huts. The nearer we drew to the beach, the more devastation we saw; eventually, only piles of rubble remained, accented by the multi-colored remnants of household belongings. Boats and boat pieces littered the landscape.

We strolled along the beach and among the rubble until we came to a concrete pad with worn red paint. In the center of what had been a front porch was a faded white design, a common talisman of greeting painted on the ground at the entrance to homes. The house was only a pile of debris with tree branches and a portion of a wall leaning against a beaten and broken form.

I was taking photos of the leaning wall when I noticed a pair of boy's shoes sitting on a built-in shelf the wall was leaning against. As I looked more closely, I realized the shoes were sitting on top of a folded jacket, pants, pack, and school slate. Next to the stack were a few small toys and a couple of painted bricks set upright with small offerings before them. Here was a shrine to a fallen boy. I reverently paused and offered prayers for the boy's family, who had clearly set this shrine here in their suffering of loss. Time stopped for just a few moments. This defamed environment now portrayed the greater destruction of the waves.

Saddened, I stepped away from the broken home. Dhamu was visiting with an elderly gentleman who had been sitting near the beach when we arrived. Vijay and Basker arrived with the customary mat and chair and placed them on the red concrete slab. I did not want to stir the spirit in this place, but it was clearly the most orderly location for us to do our work. Dhamu and the man approached me. Dhamu offered him the seat and he sat restively in its frame. Dhamu then began to recount the story he had just been told.

On the morning of December 26, this 80-year-old man had been sitting on the beach enjoying the rolling surf, which was his favorite pastime. The great wave arrived without warning and gathered him with it. He was able to grab a tree as he was being swept along and held on with all his might as the wave swallowed him and pulled with great force. He held on for as long as he could but eventually lost his struggle with the wave, let go, and disappeared into unconsciousness.

As the villagers searched the devastation later, they found his limp body amid the wreckage and, thinking him dead, took him to the temple where the rest of the dead were being gathered. At some point, someone noticed that he was still faintly breathing. They took him, teetering between life and death, to the hospital. He spent two weeks in a coma, then awakened and began to regain strength. Only a few days previous to our visit, he returned to his village and his favorite spot on the now battered beach. He reported that since awakening he had been unable to sleep, each night revisiting those horrifying moments as he clung for life. He wanted to be able to regain, along with his life, the joy he had once known on this beach.

The team gathered around him. After a grant of permission, we commenced treatment. I placed my hands on his shoulders, near the base of his neck, as Mitta took one of his hands in hers and began to gently massage it. Basker, seated at his feet, lifted a foot in his hand and began massaging also. Dhamu began his directed breathing and relaxation guidance. The man settled even deeper into the embrace of the chair, his head drifting back to rest upon my chest. I placed my hand over his heart and with Dhamu's assistance, began to guide him back to the fullness of his life.

"You are here now with us," I said. "You have survived. Your life is yours. Now rest, rest yourself here in our care and let your fears and concerns drift away."

Like a handshake or embrace we entreated one another to meet the other's need, ours to give care and his to receive. We continued the guided relaxation and release with a gentle, rhythmic pace and no thought for time. The layers of release deepened with each exhalation, his and ours.

During the treatment, a movement in the corner of my eye drew my attention away, toward the sea. I had been aware of the rolling surf since we arrived, but this wave seemed a bit taller than the rest. It seemed that it had a greater force as well. I felt a shudder within and a terror that this wave was different. This wave seemed as though it would not stop at the shore, but overwhelm the sandy beach and crash directly upon us.

Maintaining contact with the man, I turned my attention fully to the wave, responding to the inner alarm to assess our risk. Soon, I saw that the wave was shrinking. Though it was a large wave, it was not a *great* wave. It broke and rolled upon the beach as each wave before and after. In my moment of terror, however, I came to understand the fear our friends were facing. There was an innate concern that as surprising as the last, another wave would come and finish the destruction left undone. Now I began to understand this "tsunami terror". It was something inside, something anticipatory that looked for outer signals to confirm it. I exhaled, released my tension through the soles of my feet, and returned my focus to this aged infant in my hands.

We let him rest for some time. When he stirred, we helped him back to his senses, back to himself. He opened his eyes and gazed about at us with sweet kindness. He reported feeling much better, like he had a dream that he was home again, like he was back on the beach enjoying the surf. He turned to look out at the waves, took a deep breath, thanked us, and rose up from the chair.

By now several other villagers had arrived. Some reported the same conditions we had treated the previous day: bruises, sprains, cough, and "tsunami shudders". We treated them each with the same care, listening to the details of their reports and answering back with words of reassurance as we embraced them during restorative hypnotic trance. To those who presented with concerns that needed ongoing support, we instructed in the Coué Method and gave them one of the artfully prepared knotted cords. I watched with satisfaction as Dhamu recounted his instruction on emptying the stress cup each day over and over again.

One woman who complained of ongoing distress was instructed in a self-care method called 'TAT' by Mitta. It was a joy to observe Mitta demonstrating the method of placing fingers on certain regions of the face to Dhamu, who in turn demonstrated them to the woman. I was happy to sit as an observer, playing flute throughout the treatment.

Mitta and I took turns leading treatments, each according to gender and need. We observed and treated consistent complaints of the "tsunami trauma syndrome". We also repeatedly heard, upon our request for consent to treatment, that being touched by us, these caring foreigners who had come so far to be with them, was like being touched by a god.

The morning waned into early afternoon and despite the great interactions we had with the villagers, it was apparent our time for departure was at hand. We began to pack up the treatment area and gather our things when two young women appeared with a small infant, only a few months old. The mother lifted him up and toward me, saying he had a chest cold and they would like for us to give him some of the treatment we had been giving to the other villagers. In this act, the trust of a mother with her infant, I knew we had achieved success.

I received the beautiful young baby into my hands and sat gently upon the concrete slab. I heard a little congestion in his breathing, so placing him on my thighs and cradling his head in my left hand, I lowered my right hand over his chest, giving Reiki treatment to strengthen his lungs. His little eyes looked right into mine in that way little children sometimes appear to see with such deep understanding. I continued the treatment for several minutes, during which time he restfully endured this embrace from a stranger. I handed him back to the mother and thanked her, "Vanakam Nanthree."

The rest of the team was already in the vehicle when I reached it. I would have liked to spend more time with these new friends, but our schedule demanded that we move on.

After a brief stop for lunch, we returned to the work, visiting another village on our list. As we drove through the narrow streets of the village, we noted that one of the houses had a large wagon sitting in its front yard, festooned with all manner of flowers. Dhamu informed us this was an Indian hearse, that someone in this home had died and there was a funeral taking place. Our mood shifted to one of somber respect as we drove on. When we reached Dessapan's family's home, we remained in the vehicle while arrangements were made. The villagers gathered around the vehicle in a now-familiar pageant of "how do you do?" Within the group I noticed one woman who was clearly ill. Her face was drawn with pronounced cheekbones. Her eyes appeared sunken and she was thin and frail.

We climbed down from the vehicle to many greetings and were escorted into an open backyard space. Several of the villagers filed into the yard with us and soon the mat and chair were brought out. The first to take a seat in the chair was the gaunt woman I had seen in the group earlier. She appeared to have been wasting from AIDS, but when we inquired we were told that she had tuberculosis. She had been ill for some time but after the tsunami her health had dramatically declined. I was concerned about exposure. I knew that a person in this state with AIDS was at a greater risk from me than I was from her, but I did not know enough about TB transmission to know how best to protect myself and the team. I reached for my bag and retrieved the aromatic oil blend, placed a few drops in my hands, then offered the same to Mitta and Dhamu. We each inhaled the medicinal oil to give what protection we could to our lungs then turned to offer help to our new friend.

She was weak and scarcely had the strength to speak. We commenced our treatment, knowing that here our work was more palliative, giving comfort to someone who was, perhaps, approaching death. As we gave treatment, I heard what sounded like a cannon going off on the street. It was followed by the sound of a high-pitched trumpet and several other blasts. The funeral was underway. Dhamu told me that the hearse we had seen was for a victim of the tsunami who had died. As the enduring sounds of the funerary parade echoed from the street, we continued our care for this precious one still with us in the chair.

After some time of relief and strengthening, we instructed her in the Coué Method. When our treatment was complete, she arose and thanked us. She was a young woman, too young to be suffering in this way.

Two older women followed her in the chair. Each expressed similar concerns as we had treated previously and each was grateful for the relief of symptoms through our care.

During our treatment, Basker noticed a tree in the far corner of the yard. He went to the tree and began to select and cut coconuts. When we finished, he offered one to each of us, already opened and ready to enjoy. We sat together in the waning light, the villagers sitting with us, as we enjoyed our refreshing treat. The cannons and songs continued on the street, now in the distance. A flock of parrots flew overhead, chattering as they passed. The day had been long and full; our company was now ready for its own rest.

TSUNAMI EFFECT

114

18

Praying

The light was fading as we left Panietheetu. A modest temple stood at the edge of the village and beside the temple was a massive banyan tree. I requested a stop to photograph the tree and hopped from the vehicle to get a good shot. In the twilight, a good view of the tree was no longer possible, so I stepped under the low branches that reached to the ground to take some shots with flash of the majestic tree's trunk. Once inside the canopy of the tree, two male villagers directed me to a small god, wrapped in a gilded coat. The villagers asked that I take a picture of them praying before the deity and held reverent poses for the shot. We greeted one another as old friends and I felt privileged to be invited as a witness to their faith.

Dhamu arrived and told me that Mitta and the others had entered the temple and requested that I join them. The temple was an intriguingly mixed image. Set in this simple little village, high on the front of the temple was a neon sign depicting what appeared as a feather-like blade and several Tamil characters. On the ground, in front of the temple, was a stand of black spears with wide blades as their points. They were planted in the ground with the blades pointing upward in various heights and sizes. As I approached the temple, another man, about my age, welcomed me and escorted me within.

I entered an inner courtyard where a small structure stood in the middle; an austerely robed priest was at the entrance to this structure and several other villagers stood nearby. The priest entered the tiny chamber holding a platter with a flame arising from it. He waved the platter around before the deity in the tiny grotto-like structure. As he moved, shadow and light danced about the tiny nook, giving a sense of life to the entire little room. Unaware of the customs, I took my cue from those nearby, placing hands together in a prayer position and bowing my head.

My Catholic graces returned to me as I was transported to my childhood mysteries of prayers before the Crucifix and the Santos. I gave thanks for the wonderful success we had in our mission to help these villagers and others. I gave thanks for the openness of these beautiful people, for their enduring and powerful spirit that had stood throughout millennia. I asked for continued protection and guidance in our work. I stood silently in the abode of the spirit here in these different yet familiar forms and ways.

The priest emerged from the tiny chamber with the fiery platter. He held the platter before the others one at a time and I observed and repeated their practice of passing hands over the fire and carrying the smoke toward their face and over their head. This was a familiar rite from Native American ceremonies I had attended, so I, in like fashion, embraced the flame and carried its warmth and light toward me. The priest reached down toward the tray, gathered a little powder from it, and made marks upon my forehead. I accepted his benediction with humility, bowed with respect, and stepped away from the shrine threshold with the others.

What followed was something of a parade from one small niche to another. Not unlike the Stations of the Cross in the catholic liturgy, at each little alcove prayers were offered. Unfamiliar with the figures or the prayers, I simply followed the custom of the others and continued to offer my prayers of thanksgiving. We made our procession around the inner courtyard until, our prayers complete, we exited the temple where a jubilant small group was awaiting. They celebrated our attendance at their temple. They thanked us and we thanked them as we all gathered before the temple for a photograph together.

Our spirits now sated, we loaded back aboard the Cruiser and headed toward Cuddalore for the night. Cuddalore is more a large town than city, but our driver was certain there would be rooms available for us there. Upon arriving in Cuddalore and driving through the main hotel strips, his confidence began to wane.

"Uncle," Dhamodharan said, "there are many weddings taking place. We have not considered this in our planning, but we can see now that the hotels have all been filled because of all the weddings. I know it is getting late, but we will need to go back to Pondicherry to find a room for the night."

With that, we turned back onto the highway and began our thirty minute drive back to Pondi. Our hearts and minds were still full, but our bellies were beginning to feel a bit hollow. As we passed the road to Paneitheetu, from which we had recently emerged, I felt the full sense of backtracking. Continuing on, something began to feel odd about the vehicle. The driver pulled to the side of the road, climbed out, walked to the back, then came back to the front door to tell us that the rear tire had gone flat. We would all need to climb from the vehicle in order for the tire to be changed.

Darkness had fully descended, but we found a small clearing in the roadside brush with an old stone wall on which to rest and take refuge from the road. A fellow emerged from a small house near the car to offer assistance. When he saw us sitting in the nearby clearing, he insisted that we come and take rest in his house. We accepted his hospitality and entered his humble domicile. He offered us cold drinks and told us of his days in the military, showing us his ID card, now faded with age. He told us of his life working with government utility services and his pride in the work he did. We felt nurtured in his care for us needful travelers. After about twenty minutes, Vijay arrived to tell us that the car was ready to resume the trip. Our host walked us to the car and wished us safe travel as we went on our way.

When we reached Pondi, we learned to our disappointment that the Jaya Inn was full. We were fortunate to find another hotel nearby and after some wrangling over fees and passports, settled into our accommodations. It was late and we were really tired now, but food was still a vital need.

As was their custom, the men gathered and departed for a restaurant that suited their dietary needs. Mitta and I asked at the desk for a location to get vegetarian food at this late hour. The manager pointed proudly to a door adjacent to the desk.

"We have food for you here. The kitchen will close soon, but I will tell the chef to wait for your order." With that he opened the door and escorted us into a small, dimly-lit, bistro. It was smoky, and seemed more like a hotel lounge than a restaurant. The music was just a bit too loud, the light a little low, and the crowd there for drinks more than food. But after our long day, we were contented to sit, exhale, and relax with some nutrition. We reviewed the menu and ordered a plate of vegetable curry.

The waiter delivered a small tureen of well-cooked vegetables in a thick sauce. We served out portions on our small plates, tasted it, and had an immediate and simultaneous response. This was bliss. Where the Special Thali Meal had been a culinary masterpiece in many small dishes, this was the same in a single bite, with the temperature turned way up. Now almost two weeks on the ground, having sampled many fine foods, we paused to celebrate the hands-down winner of culinary mastery. What a day we had experienced; all the challenges that had brought us to this unexpected location now seemed solely for the benefit of our palates. We celebrated, bite by bite, our stumbled-upon treasure.

Our palates and bellies well-satisfied, we stepped out into the Pondi night in search of a phone center so I could call Lenise. We walked about a block from the hotel to where some men were gathered in front of a sidewalk tea stand.

"Internet?" I said, with a questioning look on my face.

The strangers looked at each other with equally quizzical glances. A tall man stepped forward. "Ah, we can see you have been to prayers tonight; for this we would like to help you. Follow this road for two blocks, turn to your left and you will see it there."

While his English was not perfect, its clarity took me by surprise; I was equally startled to remember the colored powder on my forehead. I had become accustomed to seeing the yellow marks on Mitta's forehead. We often received these blessing when visiting Dhamu's family, but in the busied events of the evening, I had forgotten my own markings.

We followed the gentleman's instruction and headed down the darkened street. It was getting late, near midnight now, and the streets took on a quiet haunting. We walked past closed shops in the still night air. We reached the end of a long block and turned. Although there were no people on the street, the small side street was populated with large oxen milling about. It seemed a rather surreal sight, amongst these quiet dusty city streets, to see a sight more familiar to a feedlot, but the oxen seemed unperturbed by our presence and continued their milling as we passed.

We could not find the browsing center, but I realized that we were near the center we had visited the night before. As we walked on and turned down the quiet street toward our destination, we heard a sound from behind us. I turned to see a small bicycle rickshaw driven by an older and withered man who looked somewhat like a Rastafarian. "Where do I need to take you?" He asked.

"We are only walking," I said, "And our destination is just ahead."

"OK," he said, "but I will see you to your stop." He continued cruising along on the street beside us. I felt a little concerned and began to map strategies in my mind of how we might defend ourselves from an attack. I stayed between Mitta and the rickshaw driver as we walked on. We exchanged names and niceties. He continued to talk with us as though we were his riders, his charge. I remained on alert, but settled comfortably into his now guardian-like presence. It was a two-block walk to the browsing center and when we arrived we parted as friends would after a journey together.

Across the telephone line, across the seas and continents from the other side of the world, I was embraced by Lenise's voice. It was like the sweet treat at the end of a full feast. I told her of our day in the villages, of our adventure in returning to Pondi, and even of the delicious curry Mitta and I had just enjoyed. She debriefed me on her day as I had on mine. We said our goodbyes across the miles. I hung up the phone. My day was complete.

Mitta and I walked back along the familiar street to the hotel. The sidewalks near the hotel were populated by street people tucked away for the night. We walked to the middle of the street and continued to take in the quiet Pondi night with each stride. As we approached the hotel, we noticed that workers had been constructing scaffolding on the street directly in front of the hotel. Even in the quiet stillness it seemed business was still under way.

Once back in my room, I settled peacefully on my bed and made some journal notes about the day. The quiet overtook me and before long I drifted serenely to sleep.

19

Drummer Boy

My hypnotherapy teacher Gil Boyne and I were visiting. A few others joined us. Gil invited us to his house for drinks. We entered a small room on the second floor, a cozy chamber that overlooked the back garden. As we laughed and celebrated being together, I began to hear a strange sound. It stirred me from my pleasant dream and filled me with a sense of dread.

On the street below, I heard the trumpet flute that was being played in the village the day before. "A funeral is going on," I thought. I arose, quickly dressed, and stepped to the landing outside my room to listen. Seeing that the sound was coming from directly in front of the hotel, I went down to investigate. Once on the street, I learned that something else altogether was going on; a wedding was taking place.

A small band with drummers and flute players paraded on the street near the now completed and colorfully decorated scaffolding in front of the hotel. I began photographing the players as we all swayed and stepped with the same rhythm. A wedding party of well-ornamented women and turban-clad men emerged from the hall adjacent to the hotel and joined in with the dance.

From around the corner, a full marching brass band in uniforms appeared, escorted by a group pushing a small cart with loudspeakers blaring music. This was the groom's procession, arriving to meet the bride for the wedding. The group arrived at the entrance to the hall and disappeared within. The band began to disperse and the wave of excitement on the street settled back to the routine swell of passing vehicles, accentuated by autorickshaw horns and bicycle bells.

I walked down the street, looking for a place to have breakfast. Down one side-street I saw a telephone booth from which I could make an international call. It was early in the morning, so I knew it would still be early evening in the States. I called my parents in Oklahoma to give them an update on my well-being and the success of our trip. They had been quite concerned about me, even though they had received my emails. Their concerns were quickly resolved and we were all delighted at the wonder of technology to speak directly from so very far away. My mother remarked on the changes since she had communicated with my father in Vietnam only through a HAM radio operator in the early '70's. We prayed together for continued safety and success and said our goodbyes.

I stepped out of the phone booth, caught in a sort of time warp and feeling each step bringing me back to the dusty road of south India. As I walked I encountered Dhamu, who was also on his way to breakfast. We walked to the hotel that had become our regular dining place. It was nice to have peaceful time with Dhamu without planning or "making arrangements". We spoke of our happiness at the success of the project, *his* project, borne of his understanding of the needs of the people who had been tsunami-affected, those living farther from his home than he had ever traveled.

While walking back after breakfast, we saw a boy, about nine years old, playing a small set of drums slung around his neck. He walked along, playing with the energy of an entire band. He paused to give us a full performance, picking up the rhythm and force just for us. We were very entertained by his vigor and drive, so we invited him back to the hotel to play for the others. There, in the hotel lobby, he rendered the same energetic delivery. We offered him rupees for his gift and he went merrily on his way, rat-tat-tatting as he did.

Before leaving Pondi for the day, there were a few details that had to be arranged. First, we went back to the Jaya Inn to reserve rooms for the evening. Next, we stopped by Western Union to retrieve funds that had been wired from the states. Mitta and I located a small homeopathic shop and purchased some remedies for those still sore and bruised or suffering from "tsunami cough".

Finally, we stopped by a shoe store. During the previous evening's escapades at the temple, Vijay had lost one of his sandals. After searching all of the racks, we found another pair of Batas like those I had purchased in Chennai. They were a little nicer than the simple sandals he had worn before, but when I saw his face shine as he saw them, I knew they were the proper replacement. I consulted with Dhamu about the sandals.

"Uncle, these will be a good pair of sandals for Vijay. They will last about four years for him."

With that report, the deal was done. Our business complete, we loaded back into the Cruiser and headed out.

Our destination was on the other side of Cuddalore, which we reached at about noon. We stopped to have our lunch, and there at the hotel we had the good fortune to meet another relief team that was working in the area. We shared time together speaking of the work we were doing in the nearby villages. Providers of material needs, they were intrigued to hear of the special service we were delivering. We departed as friends, perhaps as two fishermen passing one another and sharing reports and giving encouragement to one another.

When we reached the village of Redthiyar Pattai, it was evident that others had been there before us. At the entrance to the village, several banners promoting this and that agency were strewn across the roadway, like sponsors advertising at a sports event. It seemed a bit commercial to me, and I wondered exactly what had been provided by these groups. I turned to Mitta and suggested facetiously that perhaps we would need to purchase banners ourselves.

The crew went on their customary rounds to get permission for us to do our work. They returned with several of the villagers with them, some of whom were carrying chairs.

"Uncle, the village elders have said that they must interview you first before giving permission to work with their people. It seems many have come offering help, but have only put up signs and then left."

Mitta and I approached the small meeting area that had been set up on the other side of the banners. We were all seated in a circle and introductions were made. At first the elders seemed a bit cool to us, eyeing us with a protective suspicion. Dhamu began to explain the work that we were doing and translated the comments I made to them about what we had come to do for their people. The cool glances began to warm, and with bright Tamil smiles they welcomed us. Somehow the test and approval gave us all more confidence to approach the villagers with our gifts.

We parked the Cruiser beside a small block house. A mat and chairs were placed beneath the trees next to it and about a dozen of the villagers joined us there. One after the other brought complaints that were now very familiar: pains, coughs, and enduring fears. We followed our same pattern of providing relief through embrace and the hypnotic reset method. One after the other took their place in the chair and gave gratitude after receiving relief.

One young woman expressed her sense of loneliness while her husband was away working in another country for very long periods of time. I decided to teach her a self-care method that began with an energy meditation. I asked her to put her hands together in prayer position, the position hands would be placed to say "Namaste", or in this case, "Vanakkam". Dhamodharan continued my instruction to her, each of us sitting to either side.

"Sit quietly here for just a moment. Let yourself become perfectly still. Hear the sounds around you. Feel the gentle breeze across your face, smell the fragrances that are embracing you. Imagine all of these as a source of your strength. In this stillness, allow this strength to flow through you, and to gather between your hands like a warm and glowing ball. Let this ball begin to expand and grow, causing your hands to drift apart. Continue to experience the beauty that is around you and continue to allow that beauty to move through you and collect and grow between your hands, causing them to move farther and farther apart."

As she settled, a quiet grace washed over her face. Her body relaxed, her breathing eased, and her hands moved apart slowly. I felt, again, the privilege of being present to the effects of a great spirit of healing.

"Now bring those hands, rich with your own strength, with palms facing you, toward your face, your throat, your heart. Feel the same presence of calm and beauty now radiating from all around you, through you, and back to you again. Remember this feeling, remember this ability, and draw on this for your strength and comfort at any time you need."

She settled back into the chair, so passive and peaceful after her earlier presentation of distress. In time she opened her eyes, looked about at those of us so tenderly focused on her well-being, and gave a radiant smile. She brought her hands back again to the same prayer position, and as was a familiar custom, she bowed toward us and said "Nanthree, thank you."

We, in turn, repeated the same.

As she arose from the chair the daylight was fading; no shadows remained. In this encroaching twilight the mosquitos, called "cusos" in Tamil, made their assault. We fled for the Cruiser to gather our spray repellent and decided that we must conclude our clinic. There were still several waiting for treatments, so we called those who were in need to come to the Cruiser where we distributed swabs saturated with the aromatic lung medicines to each of them. When I had finished with the line of villagers, darkness was upon us. I went back to the site of the open-air clinic and found Dhamu there, surrounded by about half a dozen villagers, all standing and attending his instruction.

Dhamu stood confidently before the group of elder women and men, demonstrating the lesson of "emptying the stress cup". He held his cupped hand up and with the other demonstrated the flow of burden into the cup, then turned the cup to empty its contents and restore calm. I did not know a single word he spoke, but my heart heard him saying. "It is most important that you empty this cup each day to secure your well-being."

I called Mitta toward me to witness the display. We both stood in silence together. The student and facilitator had truly become the teacher, a leader for his people.

20

Parade

It was nice to be back in Pondicherry for the night. It had become a familiar and homey place, and the Jaya Inn provided a nice spot for us to rest and recover from a full day in the field. After a delicious dinner, we were fortunate, with some inquiry, to find a music shop where I was able to purchase a flute like the one I had heard that morning. The shopkeeper was impressed that I could, after only hearing it a bit, produce a string of notes from the double-reed, oboe-like instrument. I learned that it was called a "nathaswaram", and was traditionally used in parades.

The next morning I arose to a commotion within the group. Dhamu had been contacted by his mother and informed that a census was to take place in Srinivasapuram. Everyone would need to be present by early afternoon or risk being underserved in government relief efforts. Though we had planned on outreach in more villages, we would have to hurry back to Chennai.

We loaded our bags and stopped for breakfast at our familiar hotel. We had finished our standard breakfast of idli and omelet and were just savoring our last minutes in Pondi when our attention was drawn to some activity out on the street. Horns were honking more than usual, and another kind of bell ringing, drum beating, and jubilation of many voices seemed to be causing a stir.

We emerged from the restaurant and beheld a true spectacle. Out on the street a parade was taking place. Loud drums reverberated throughout the area. A marching band in brilliant blue uniforms with tufted turbans led the procession. Behind them, beautifully ornamented wagons pulled by tractors carried a variety of riders in all manner of gilded attire. Horses and Brahma bulls, covered with ornate shroud-like blankets, followed. A lumbering elephant similarly adorned and escorted by celebrants, elevated the parade to a pageant. This entourage was followed by a column of young women in every color of shimmering saris. The music continued as the procession passed and one of the attendants stopped to inform me that a new temple was opening and this was the celebration to mark its new beginning.

Only minutes after the great swell had begun, it passed, and the street returned to its normal level of human clamor. We climbed inside the Cruiser and commenced our own parade of departure from Pondicherry. Now the stone pillars that divided the Pondicherry French province from greater Tamil Nadu seemed like a gateway out of the Emerald City, out of the mystique of the villages and the great Tamil spirits who had shown us their simple and majestic ways, out of a dream-like destiny of different worlds embracing one another.

The mood in the car was one of deflation. There was more we wanted to do. Beyond Cuddalore lay Nagapatinum, the most severely tsunami-affected area. We had conceded earlier that we would not reach this area, but every village nearer seemed a closer reach that we must now release. We watched the passing fields and passersby on the road with a certain melancholy. We were satisfied beyond expectations at our success, but still longed to do more.

Mitta commented that she had misplaced a bracelet and thought perhaps she had left it at the hotel in Mamallapuram. As it was a brief detour to go into the village and check, we found ourselves back in the travelers' district of this ancient destination. Here was our accommodation, the Sakthi Guest House, and we stepped inside to inquire whether the bracelet had been found.

As Mitta and the attendant went upstairs to check the room, my attention was drawn to a poster on the wall I had overlooked during our stay. The poster depicted an impressionist view of a Tamil village. Below the image were the words "What we learn with pleasure we never forget". I stood before the poster as all the flavors and emotions floated back to me. They rested on my palate and settled in my heart. Like the poster, many of the events of the preceding days had flashed by as they occurred, as we were immersed in planning and implementing. Now, having completed the work, the delight and reward resonated with me. The dusty, dank smell of the old hotel wrapped around me and sealed the feeling within.

I stepped out onto the roadway and was instantly approached by two young girls selling beaded strands. They seemed like sisters and worked the tourists well, one nodding to lower prices while the other conservatively demanding a firm price. We settled between the two and I felt as happy to have the trinkets as to have participated in a family tradition. As we departed Mamallapuram, I looked back and saw that the guys in the back were letting their eyes linger behind as well. This too was a place we felt forced to pry ourselves from, hoping to one day return, but trying, somehow, to bring a bit of it with us.

It was just past noon when we arrived at the outskirts of Chennai. A sudden sense of culture shock came over me. I turned to Mitta to discuss this feeling that even though we had only been on the trip for a few days, it seemed that we had entered another world altogether. We had entered a part of India that few travelers would find. We had sat in sorrow with the people in these places and had been brought into their lives. It was a gift, a treasure, a true odyssey of hope and blessings. Perhaps, we thought, we had seen a part of India that even many Indians, particularly those living in the congested cities like Chennai, would find foreign as well.

The multi-colored shops and vendors lining the streets of Adyar closed around us as we were immersed again into the city. The faces on the street seemed dull and distracted, numbly trapped in the routines of their lives. What had before seemed exotic, now appeared mundane, the ongoing common rites of everyday life. We arrived in Srinivasapuram to the same sense of diminishing expectancy. The guys checked in with family members and we continued on to Mylapore in search of accommodations.

There were no rooms available at the MGM Grand, so we traveled on to other hotels Dhamu had surveyed before our arrival in India. We checked several before settling in at the Ram Guest House in Royapetta. The area was a little more congested than where we had been in Mylapore, but the long driveway that led to the hotel gave us a sense of seclusion. It was a recently constructed three-story structure, clean and smelling of fresh paint. Mitta and I settled in to our rooms and Dhamu returned to his own home after making arrangements to pick us up for dinner in a few hours.

After resting for about an hour, Mitta and I went out to survey our new neighborhood and locate the nearest browsing center. Adjacent to the end of the drive, right on the narrow sidewalk near the road, was a small tea stand. We stood gawking as the attendant prepared the tea by ladling a small portion from a sunken pot into a small metal cup, then pouring from one cup to another repeatedly as he drew the cups farther apart, at times causing the cascading tea to fall over two feet into the lower cup. It was a wonderful spectacle to observe, like the tossing of a pizza crust, but served the purpose of cooling somewhat while adding froth to the tea. Though I was still pleasantly abstaining from caffeine, Mitta was thrilled to enjoy a cup of the tea and made fast friends with the attendants who would become her most frequent encounters in the coming days.

Across the street was a small hospital with a banner in the front promoting Yoga classes. Along the street beside the hospital was a small sign announcing our sought-after browsing center. We crossed the road, only to find that the center was not yet open. Upon inquiry, we learned there was an open center about one mile away, so we set out to discover it and to learn more of our new domain. Though this area was more congested than the one we had previously stayed in, being a Saturday afternoon, there was a lazy, sauntering rhythm on the street. As we passed by a contemporary western hotel, I noticed a small sign offering Reiki at a nearby clinic. Further down the road we discovered a Pizza Hut and happily sat to enjoy a familiar taste of home.

With some continued searching, we found the browsing center we had set out for and entered the small office building, took the elevator to the basement, and arrived to find the staff struggling to reboot the entire system after a power outage. Our patience prevailed and we were soon satisfied to have checked in with our community at home.

We continued to explore our new neighborhood, finding just the right restaurant to enjoy our next meals and purchasing some bananas from a street vendor as the afternoon winter light began to grow golden and cool. We walked down the street beyond the browsing center and hospital to find a nice residential area with comfortable small homes similar to my neighborhood in Venice Beach. People were about their common affairs and I felt a sort of belonging unlike that I had experienced in any district we had yet encountered.

We turned a corner and discovered, with mysterious awe, a small temple, not much larger than a two car garage, nestled in the middle of the neighborhood. This temple stood out among all the other temples we had seen in India or Singapore. Those had been painted in bright colors with the figurines that ensconced the roof painted in realistic hues with gilded attire. This temple was completely white, as though the whole thing had been carved from the purest marble or alabaster. A majestic serenity exuded from it. In this quiet place, all alone, as though it had been delivered there just for the refreshment of our own spirits, this small temple stood peacefully in the still, warm, early evening light. There was nothing left for us on this excursion but to simply take it in and return to our hotel to prepare for our evening appointment with Dhamodharan.

21

Family

When leaving us earlier in the day, Dhamu had told us he had something special to share with us and he would return in the early evening. When he arrived to gather us, he would only say that there was someone important that he wanted us to meet. We climbed into the Cruiser and set out on an adventure in the Chennai night. A new, more modern electric city revealed itself. Vibrant billboards presented contemporary clothing and perfume advertisements. Steel and glass storefronts displayed the financial and commercial strength of the area. As we turned down one street, we noticed a wide window display of coffins and other funerary items. Such a public and ornate display was perhaps one of the most foreign observations I had made; coffins and other elements of the rites of death were not part of my American motif.

We arrived at last at our destination and entered a non-descript building, something like a small apartment building, climbing stairs to a second-floor room where we were introduced to Dhamu's friend KS Mohideen. We climbed another flight of stairs to a rooftop and I realized this was not an apartment building, but a multistoried home, strangely configured into individual living spaces. The rooftop space was simple, but looked out over the bustling city; the sounds of the night were calmer, but still as dense as those during the day. The coolness of the air invited an embrace of city and sky.

Dhamodharan pointed to a small room in the corner of the rooftop, about six by eight feet in size. "Here," he said. "This is where my family came to live when we were saved from our desperate situation sleeping for days on the sidewalk. My friend was very kind to give us this space as shelter."

We stepped into the tiny room, barely the three of us fitting within. Dhamu stood near one corner. The dim light evoked the sorrow and sense of desperation that he and the other nine members of his family had felt until the day we arrived in Chennai. There was both sadness and celebration: an understanding of how very difficult things had been for the family, yet the knowledge of how this family had given support to Dhamodharan's, helping them to regain their wave-robbed dignity.

Mitta and I both offered thankfulness to Dhamu's friend as his friend's mother now joined us on the rooftop. She greeted us briefly, departed, and soon returned with trays full of familiar and delicious foods: idli, dosa, sambar, and channa masala. A plastic mat was spread out and we sat together to enjoy the feast of friendship and fine food. We spoke of the work we had been doing in India, of how that work was born of a greater mission to reduce suffering worldwide, and how it had all begun through the efforts to help people with AIDS die more graciously. We found that this was a shared mission, as his friend was working in AIDS hospice services as a social worker. Tale-by-tale and bite-by-bite, the evening drifted. Reluctantly, we said our goodbyes and returned to our accommodations at the Ram Guest House for the night.

We agreed to a noon rendezvous, so I took Sunday morning to myself to catch up on notes and organizational concerns. The television in my room presented mostly channels broadcasting Bollywood-styled dance videos. I had termed them "cooing videos" due to the universal plot of the guy trying to get the girl who always coyly retreated from his boisterous and amorous advances. I was delighted to find a channel broadcasting a program in English titled *University Challenge*. This quiz show featured teams of university students working against others. To my good fortune, I had caught the finals and was impressed by the intellect of the students. Special guest Ravi Shankar presented the trophy to the champions and eloquently expressed my own thoughts on the brilliance of all the participants.

Dhamu and Vijay arrived according to schedule. We fetched Mitta and made our way to Srinivasapuram. The village was more subdued than the day before. Trucks had come to collect piles of debris gathered from the tsunami destruction and a feeling of transformation resonated on the street. We walked down the familiar pathway toward Vijay's destroyed home. Beside the remaining rubble, a makeshift shelter had been erected: a salvaged sale banner stretched as a canopy, anchored to a denuded tree and tied off to several bamboo poles standing in the sand with bricks and stones propping them upright.

The midday sun bore down, cooking the air and making the sand too hot to stand on in bare feet. Beneath the shaded canopy sat an old wooden crate and a bundle of fishing nets. Several of the village men had gathered, perhaps to help with our efforts, perhaps simply in anticipation of observing the work we had come to do. A mat and chair were brought out and set up in a now standard rite of commencement. Several village women approached and, as we had many times before, we invited any in need to take a place in the chair and receive care.

One by one several women took their place in the chair. We listened to their reports and shared their sorrow and sense of dismay at the challenges they were facing in restoring their disrupted lives. We quickly decided what methods and which therapist would work where and in what way. We then reached out our hands, took them into our care, and set about helping them to put things straight within their hearts and minds.

In time, a young girl about ten years old took her place in the chair as her mother sat by expressing her concern. The young girl, we were told, could not find any happiness. While all the other children seemed contented to run and play, even upon the rubble of former homes, she wore a mask of sadness, of withdrawal, of reticence to even enter the game of life. Mitta guided the treatment, reaching out to take her hand from a kneeling position before her, looking into her eyes with kindness, and softly saying, "It's OK, I understand. Life can be so troubling at times, seeming to be more than we can even bear. There is much in life to be glad for, much to help give us happiness, to help wash our sadness away."

The young girl looked back at Mitta, her eyes becoming a little more focused and bright, as small movements began to transform her paralytic mouth into the first impressions of a smile. Now what began in the eyes and traveled to the mouth moved across the whole face as her skin took on a new glow, the light of hopefulness. As Mitta instructed her to close her eyes and relax into the chair, the entire team reached out to rest hands upon her shoulders and feet as she was guided to release her sorrow and recall pleasant, even happy times in her life. Small tears began to run from the corner of her eyes while a slump of acceptance revealed her surrender to the possibility of some greater potential for her life.

Throughout the treatment her mother sat attentively, observing her daughter's transformation and the methods we were using to give her care. When the treatment was complete, the daughter stood from the chair, looked lovingly at Mitta, and gave her the embrace one would a family member, holding her as if to retain the full benefit of their time together.

The seat now empty, the mother rose from her corner under the shade canopy and took her place in the chair. It seemed as though the time with her daughter was a test to see if we were capable of actually helping her.

As she settled in the chair, she informed us that she had been trapped in sorrow for a very long time. She reported that her life had been such a challenge to be alone and raising a child, that she felt lost. Her tears erupted and she confessed that even before the tsunami she had felt compelled to simply walk into the sea and vanish. This report gave us more understanding as to the despair the daughter had developed, experiencing the collateral impact of her mother's suffering.

With practiced precision, the team went to work. We placed hands upon her as I took my position standing over the chair, my own hands on her shoulder and side of her head. We commenced our relaxation routine, guiding her to release tension from head to toe as we massaged hands and feet. "Release your sadness and pain, be free now, we are here with you giving you care; you are not alone."

She let out a crying moan, seeming to release herself from her own body, which now collapsed in the chair and cascaded like water from the chair onto the ground. She whimpered as she lay there, the team responding to her movement, maintaining contact and helping her to settle comfortably on the shaded sand.

Now her own mother stirred compassionately from her place and reached out to join our caring embrace of her daughter. Her hands resonated in a way ours could not, nearly trembling with the drive to answer the eminent needs of her daughter. As her hands settled, the woman's body responded to the touch that only one could give her, the loving touch of a mother that a child can distinguish in a mob. The mother looked at me for consent, now realizing she had acted on impulse. I smiled, holding back my own torrent of tears.

I looked around at several other women sitting around the circle whose eyes also asked, "May I?" With my nod they all reached out to put hands upon her as I continued "You are surrounded with love now. You are in the hands of family and community, those who are with you now and always to give you strength when you need it, to help you to carry your burdens, to participate in the goodness you come to know each day. Let your body, your mind, your heart, now know that this love is true, that it is always there. See yourself in the future; know this truth of the love around you, toward you, for you. Let this knowledge be as a force within you, helping you in all ways."

I'm not sure how Dhamu translated my words, but as he spoke she continued to settle deeper and deeper upon the ground as all hands gently swayed her body with a reinforcing sense of comfort, like rocking a baby. What had been a storm now settled into stillness. We all experienced a deep and restive sigh as in the quiet, I informed her to take her time and awaken as though from a true dream when she was ready.

After some moments, she reported that her eyes were stuck closed and she needed someone to put water on her face so she could open them. There was a glass of water sitting nearby. I picked it up and handed it to her mother who was sitting nearest to her face. As I was looking about for a cloth to moisten in the water, I observed with surprise that her mother simply reached her hand into the glass, scooped out a handful of water, and thrust it into her daughter's face. With near slow motion detail, I watched the hand-sized pond drifting and spilling across the arm's reach explode and scatter as it hit her face. I was astonished and thought what a disruptive finish it was to such a sedating intervention, but as the woman's hand rose to remove the drench from her face, her eyes opened and she looked up with gratitude to first her mother, then the team, then the rest of the villagers who had gifted her with a sense of her own worth.

After the treatment we sat together for some time, just appreciating being together as stories were told back in forth. Looking out upon the sea, Dhamu commented "Uncle, you have been very happy with the help that Vijay has given on this project, but you must know that his true strength is on the sea. There he is like a king."

"Then we must go to sea together" I responded.

Dhamu and Vijay spoke back and forth as they looked out upon the water. Some of the other men chimed in on the conversation. "Uncle, they say that Tuesday will be a good day to go to sea.

"Then on Tuesday," I said, "we must allow Captain Vijay to take us out."

"I will make the arrangements, Uncle."

Our work in the village complete for the day, we headed back to the Ram Guest House for the night. My curiosity about the yoga classes advertised at the small hospital across the street compelled me to go inquire about details. I entered the three-story building that was open, though nearly vacant, as it was Sunday. Once inside I asked for more information about the yoga classes advertised. I was informed that the instructor was not present, but if I would leave my name and some manner of contact, she would be notified. I left my name and told them that I was a guest across the street.

The day was now fading but one important task still lay ahead. We had been invited to a wedding that was scheduled at six o-clock the following morning. Dhamu had explained that weddings were scheduled for the most astrologically auspicious time and in this case that meant the crack of dawn. It would take at least an hour to travel the distance, so we set our pickup time for 4:45. It would be necessary to take a gift for the bride and groom, so Mitta and I set out for a shop to find an appropriate item for a new couple's household.

We had already discovered a nice American Hotel restaurant about two blocks from the Ram Guest House; we noticed a gift shop across the street as we were arriving for dinner. We entered the shop and discovered all manner of items perfect for a fresh young couple. After shopping for some time, we settled on a joint purchase of a nice lamp with built-in clock. We were doubly delighted that the shop also offered gift-wrapping. Our errands complete, we strolled back to our rooms to settle in for an early evening in preparation for a very early morning ahead.

22

Love Day

St. Valentine's Day has always been a special holiday for Lenise and me. For the first time in twenty-one years we would be spending the day apart, half a world away from each other. To compound the circumstance, on this day we were to attend our first Tamil wedding, an event I could not fully celebrate without my valentine.

Our day began long before the dawn. I arose before 4:00 am and thought it seemed a very strange time to go to a wedding. I have always enjoyed rising at such a time, as it recalls fond memories of rising early to go fishing with my father. There is a quiet excitement that stirs within me in these early hours, as though the full potential for the day can truly be realized. I find it similar to that feeling of arriving at the theater hours before the show, to be a witness to the greater drama of an unfolding event.

Mitta and I met at the hotel desk at 4:30 to be ready for Dhamodharan's arrival at 4:45. By 5 he had still not arrived and I began to grow anxious. At 5:15 I decided to take action. I showed the invitation to the desk clerk and asked for help. Together we went to the street and stopped an autorickshaw. Assuring us he could deliver us to the distant destination on time if we departed immediately, we climbed into the back of the tiny chariot and set out in the cold Chennai darkness.

The customarily open carriage was now closed with black and clear plastic encasement, much like that of a jeep soft-top. Though it blocked most of the incoming air, the chill of the breeze as we blasted through the streets at the little vehicle's top speed pierced the shroud and caused us to brace ourselves as we also leaned forward with the anticipation of reaching the wedding on time.

We crossed a great bridge and the city lights danced all about us, off to such a far away location with no guide, only trust and hope. After what seemed as though it would be an endless drive, we pulled up before a group of buildings. The driver called out to a fellow who was standing in front, and after an exchange of words and gestures, we were on our way again.

We seemed to drive again for about the same distance and it was now after 6:00 as we pulled up to another nondescript and seemingly deserted building. The driver assured us we were at the address on the paper. As we stepped out of the auto and paid him our fare, I could hear some music in the adjacent building.

The light within warded off the shadows of the street, just as the walls offered warmth from the cool early morning air. We followed individuals down a hallway to what seemed to be the meeting room for the wedding as their eyes studied our foreign appearance. While we were still in the hallway, we heard a commotion at the door and turned to see a large entourage entering the building. A priest accompanied them, clad only in a wrinkled white lungi with a soiled towel over his shoulder and streaks of yellow powder across his head. Thin white hair cascaded from his balding head and he appeared to have already put in a day's work.

The groom followed, dressed in fresh white lungi and shirt with a white turban and a grand garland of white, pink, and green flowers hanging heavily around his neck. A friend stood by holding an umbrella over him, though there was no rain. A plastic chair was placed in the middle of the hallway and the groom took his seat there, surrounded by women in beautiful, multi-colored saris and several children, also dressed in fine clothes. As he sat, two silver trays were placed by his feet, one empty and one containing a coconut, banana, incense, and numerous other leaves and herbs.

The priest placed a small piece of gel on the floor and set it aflame as he kneeled at the groom's feet and began to chant. He cracked the coconut on the floor and allowed the milk to pour out over the groom's feet, which had been placed in the empty tray. As he continued to chant, he lifted this substance, then that substance from the tray and placed them on the groom's feet. He appeared not to just be blessing, but also seeking signs in the various elements in the tray. He spoke to the groom reassuringly as the onlookers seemed to accept some good report. The umbrella replaced over the groom's head, he stood and the whole company made their way to the meeting room, as we followed behind.

The room was dim, illuminated only by the half-lit bulbs that were further occluded by many paper decorations hanging from the ceiling, and a thin fog of smoke. On a platform, several musicians sat playing drums and large flute-like instruments, similar to the nathaswaram parade flute, but much larger. About forty people were already sitting in the arranged chairs, ready for the ceremony to begin, as we took our seats near the back of the group.

Moments later the groom's father, whom we recognized from his visit to offer his invitation, arrived to greet us. He insisted that we take a seat of honor on the front row and escorted us there. As we took our new seats the ceremony got under way on a platform stage before us. The area had been decorated with a frame built around an area about ten by ten feet. It was draped with many orange, yellow, and white flower garlands that obscured the mural of a Hindu deity on the wall behind it.

Within the frame, the floor was covered with many clay pots, some stacked on one another, towers of oil lamps, and many different flowers and powders arranged on large banana leaves that were laid out like a carpet. As the bride and groom gathered within the frame, many other celebrants that I assumed to be family members stood around them. As I began to snap photos, a gentleman approached me and invited me to come up to the platform to take my photographs. From this advantage I could see the ceremony much more clearly.

The bride and groom took seats on the floor beneath the frame and a small tray of water and powders was placed before the groom. The groom's parents stepped forward, placing their feet in the tray. Some of the surrounding celebrants steadied them. The groom began to lift water from the tray with his hand and pour it over their feet, applying different powders as he did. After some minutes, the parents stepped from the tray onto a pad to absorb the water from their feet. The bride's parents took their turn in another tray before the bride as she repeated the ritual, the washing and blessing of the feet.

The drums and horns continue their long song. A tray filled with some plant material was placed before the bride and groom and the material was set on fire. As the fire blazed, smoke danced up from the tray and filled the entire frame area, enveloping us all in its cloud. The priest gave a small bottle to the groom as he continued his chanting. He instructed the groom to use the small scoop to apply the liquid to the fire. As the liquid cascaded onto the flames, they jumped higher, giving another burst of smoke. The priest chanted louder and more intently as he encouraged the groom to continue his actions with what I now assumed to be oil. Another tray that contained a coconut resting on a bed of rice and ornamented with the same red and yellow flowers and powders was set beside the flaming, smoking tray.

Some of the celebrants stepped forward and began to attend to the bride. They draped gold chains over her neck, and then began placing gold ornaments with strings attached to her forehead. They carefully centered the piece over her forehead and gathered the strings to tie them from behind. Several individuals in succession applied the ornaments, and then began to do the same for the groom. The priest's chants bellowed like the smoke, joining the ongoing music, stirring my mind and lifting me like an autumn leaf in a breeze, caught up in a rapturous event.

After further attention was given to the tray with the coconut, it was taken from the platform by one of the priest's young assistants and carried around the room. Each of the attendees touched the coconut with a blessing and gathered a small portion of the rice. The coconut tray was brought back to the platform and the coconut was placed in the bride's lap. A piece of fabric was wrapped around it and her, suggesting a pregnant belly. More chants and blessings were made, now particularly toward the bride, in what seemed to be a fertility rite within the marriage ceremony. With a shout, the entire company threw the rice they had gathered toward the bride and groom. The coconut was then removed from the drape and placed back in its tray.

Next, the bride rose from her seat, along with the groom, and the two of them walked to one side of the frame. There a flat stone used for grinding grain sat with its cylindrical pestle resting on top of it. The bride placed her foot on the stone and the groom bent down to place a small golden ring on her second toe. With this act, the ceremony was complete. More rice was thrown and the priest concluded his incantations. Congratulatory greetings were made between the bride and groom and their parties.

I heard a voice behind me. It was Dhamodharan. "Uncle, I am so glad to see that you are here. When I could not find you at the hotel I was concerned, but I see that you were able to make it here on your own."

"We had help from our driver and quite a ride getting here as well. Have you only just arrived?"

"No Uncle, we came in during the marriage but I did not want to interrupt you during your photography."

As we were speaking, I noticed that sparkling stainless steel bowls and buckets were being brought out from a door beside the platform and placed on the floor between the platform and the guest seating. Then, with industrial precision, a great array of all manner of household vessels and utensils was spread out on the floor before me. There were trays holding small piles of folded fabric with small clusters of baby bananas atop them.

I turned quizzically to Dhamodharan. "It is dowry, Uncle."

I continued to watch and photograph as family members exchanged gifts of cloth with each other, Dhamodharan explaining the custom and relationships. The cloth that was presented to the groom had been tailored into an exquisite business shirt. By now the music had stopped and many of the guests had left the room. I began to interact with several of the children who were lingering for the gifting session. After a brief absence, the groom returned dressed in black slacks and his new grey shirt, the gold ornaments still tied around his head, looking like the king on his day of coronation. He joined us to thank us for attending and we gave him our own gift for their new home.

"Uncle we must go eat now" Dhamodharan said as he escorted us out of the large room, through a hallway, and down a flight of stairs to a banquet hall one floor below. We entered a large room with tables laid out in long rows that ran the length of the hall. There were plastic chairs set on one side of the table. The room was about half-filled with celebrants, so we wasted no time in finding a place to sit.

As soon as we sat, a fellow passed by and placed a banana leaf on the table before us. No sooner had the leaf rested upon the table than a brigade of bucket-bearing servers paraded past, depositing all manner of treat before us: sweet grain pastes, idli, and vada, a seasoned fried donut that, dipped in the accompanying coconut chutney, was divine. The servers kept a pace along the tables and anytime a vacancy appeared on the leaf, an offering was made. The cavalcade of flavors accentuated the grand pageant of love, family, and community.

"Uncle, there is something very important I must show you. When you have completed your meal, it is important that you let them know by folding your leaf closed. If the leaf is folded toward the servers it will be an insult, a rejection. But if it is folded toward you, it will say that 'I am with you.' You must fold your leaf toward you when you have finished." With that, he folded his leaf closed. Mitta and I both folded ours in the similar manner as we rose from the table to begin our trek back to the hotel.

We arrived back at the Ram Guest House just before noon. Mitta was scheduled to return to the states on the following evening. After a few hours spent resting, packing, and checking in at the browsing center that had now opened across the street, we set out to purchase some souvenir items for her to take home. Since she wanted a couple of nice saris, Dhamodharan said he knew the perfect place to shop. He took us to a beautiful temple center that we had previously seen when driving through the neighborhoods near the MGM Grand Hotel. The temple was multi-tiered with gilded objects and painted figures adorning each level as it rose up toward heaven. Around the temple square were vendor booths selling all manner of collectable trinkets. I was thrilled to find a small plastic flute with keys like tiny piano keys, called a "melodica". A toy instrument in reality, it still produced good tones and would complement the other toy instruments in my collection. Mitta and I walked on as Dhamu negotiated a fair price.

Across the road from the vendor booths were the permanent shops that sold "puja" materials for ceremonies. I browsed in shops for a small bell, while Mitta went looking for saris. After a sufficient period of shopping, and having acquired adequate treasure for her return home, Mitta and I turned our attention to one further purchase. Together, we had already conferred with Jim Uncle and decided to pool our funds to purchase a special "thank you" gift for Dhamodharan. He had informed us of the importance of having a nice wristwatch for his approaching employment. We told him of our scheme and asked for his advice on the appropriate shop. He knew just the place to go.

After perusing a few of the vendors along the way, we wound through the neighboring streets of the temple plaza and arrived at a nice shop that sold only watches. With determined precision, Dhamu went from this counter to the next, assessing this feature then that. Within the complex were two other watch shops, so we diligently searched every rack in each shop. At long last, Dhamodharan made his selection. We happily made our purchase and observed the look of pride as he placed the shiny new timepiece on his wrist. With this one act he also seemed to don the manner and presence of a professional.

Our next stop would prove to be even more transformational. The sun was going down and we were all a bit ready for a rest. We noticed a small restaurant/bar and decided to take a break. At first, Dhamu said that he would be happy to wait for us outside as we went in to enjoy a beverage and a snack. After some insistence on our part, he relented to join us. It was a western-styled bar and as we entered, his tension increased. "Uncle, you must know that I would never be able to enter this place if I were not with you."

The waiter deposited a bowl of crunchy snacks before us as we ordered a couple of beers and a soda for Dhamu. He refused alcohol for he had shown us the small open-shed "wine shops" in the villages and told us how the alcohol sold there was very strong and destroyed men's lives and families. We comfortably sat, enjoying our beverages and snacking on the mix of nuts and seasoned, fried noodle bits. It had been a long day and it felt good to be in a near-western environment on plush sofas. I began to understand, however, that this little stop revealed the remaining divisions of race, class, and culture that separated our worlds. We were all happy to step back onto the street and continue our trek home.

The Ram Guest House was close, so we decided to walk the distance. Along the way we encountered a small street bazaar with many vendors proffering their goods on blankets laid out on the road. I perused the blankets and found a small drawing of Ganesha, the elephant god, depicted through many different leaves as body parts. It was very charming, particularly because the leaves were "elephant ear" leaves and it reminded me of the magnificent plant Lenise had grown in the garden in Venice and made me feel a bit of home. I turned the board over and was astonished to see a partial sticker across the back reading "Tucumcari Tonite". Below that it also said "Serving you on Rt 66 for 70 years".

Tucumcari, New Mexico is a well-known stopover on Rt66/I-40. Though Lenise and I have been through there dozens of times on our jaunts between LA and OKC, I first remember Tucumcari from my earliest childhood, as it was the turnoff to the family ranch in the Oklahoma panhandle. When traveling with my family from California, it meant we were almost to the paradise called the Anchor D Ranch. Standing here, in this far away place, holding an object with such distant and familiar images made the whole world seem to close about me, not like a crush, but an embrace.

We walked on through the dark and dusty streets, eventually arriving back at the hotel. Mitta went to her room and Dhamu and I hopped on his two-wheeler to ride to the browsing center. It was getting late. When we arrived at the browsing center, some of the street dwellers were already bedding down on the walkways near the center. I entered the brightly lit room and went to a calling booth, dialed automatically, and waited longingly for the voice to answer on the other end. Lenise picked up the line and greeted me from around the world.

"Happy Valentine's Day, my love."

23

To Sea

We arrived in Srinivasapuram at mid-morning, walking our familiar trail to the beach through the narrow alleyway, past the decimated rubble of Vijay's house and the humble tarp canopy that had served as our treatment clinic. As we walked onto the beach, it appeared as it had not until this time. Where previously the beach had been empty except for dotted shelters, now it was adorned with various fishing boats: long open-hulled fiberglass boats and wood-beam kattumarams. Bundles of nets lay beside the boats, being tended by the men with assistance from several women. Dhamu guided us to a boat beside which Vijay was completing his rolling of nets. An older woman was stooping down to pick up fish from the sand and place them in an age-worn tub. There was an exhilarating sense of possibility reverberating along the beach.

Upon our arrival, Vijay conferred with several of the other men tending to their nets. Together, they began to survey a nearby boat, making gestures and comments as they did. Two men approached with long rough wooden poles and began to place the poles through ropes attached to the side of the boat. One group set the pole at the rear of the boat as another began to do the same near the front of the boat. In time, they had succeeded in securing the poles through the ropes across the width of the boat. Several other men approached as Vijay, with his Sequoia-like stature, braced one end of a pole across his stout shoulders, guiding the others to do the same. As these strongmen took control of the poles, several others, Dhamu and me included, took positions at the rear of the boat. With a shout the poles were lifted, bringing the boat slightly from its nest in the sand as we all thrust forward to scoot the massive vessel along the sand to the surf's edge. Two others approached with a similar pole bearing a large gas-powered motor that had a five-foot long shaft with a propeller at the end. The motor was attached to the rear of the boat and secured in place, propeller suspended above the water.

The boat, now slightly afloat in the rolling surf, was maneuvered to face the sea as those of us who had helped to convey it from the sand waded out and climbed over the sturdy side rails to find our place within. Several others stood at the waterline and waved their wishes toward us as the boat drifted out upon the water.

Vijay climbed onto the back of the boat, took a small cord attached to the motor and, wrapping it securely around a disc on the top of the motor, gave it a swift pull, sending the motor into a raging roar. His other hand firmly on the tiller bar protruding from the motor, he lowered the whirring propeller into the water; the boat lurched forward, raising its nose above the oncoming waves. We bounced over the series of rolling waves and found ourselves beyond the breaks, motoring out to sea with Captain Vijay at the helm.

Mitta, Dhamu, and I had taken our places on the floor of the boat as the two other fishermen who accompanied us picked up spooled lines with lures attached. Casting the lures into the sea, they rolled out a length of line and tied it securely to their ankle in the hopes of catching some fish along the way.

The speed of the boat seemed to increase even more. The nose of the twenty-five-foot craft rose further upward as though we would take flight above the sea. Mist sprayed from every direction, dousing us with the fine taste of salty air. I looked back to see Vijay, standing proud like the most ancient of mariners, his bare feet grasping the rail of the end of the boat, his hand firmly guiding the tiller and his eyes cast out far upon the waters, seeing the unseen, a master at his craft with the fullness of his unconquerable majesty.

As we cruised along the water, the shoreline began to fade in the distance. One of the fishermen rose from his seat on the outer rail and walked to the middle of the open boat, picked up a rope that was tethered to the front of the boat and stood in the same manner as Vijay, his feet planted firmly, his eyes outwardly cast, his hand grasping the rope like a charioteer's reins. We chuckled in amusement at this image and were invited to take his place. Mitta went first, rising from her seat to take hold of the rope and, using it to pull herself up to her feet, now stood firmly in a wide stance. After some time, she turned and offered the rope to me.

I rose in similar manner, took the rope in hand and felt my feet anchor me, as though magnetized to the floor of the boat. The sea opened more fully around me. I was riding upon the water now, as the boat continued its steady rise and fall over the tops of small waves. I leaned back hard against the rope and yielded to my sense of flight. Feeling the strength in my legs and the absence of need for security, I loosened the tension on the rope and let it drop like slack reins. Now, only my feet and balance kept me at my stance, causing me to feel as though I was surfing the sea on this great craft, a strangely exhilarating inner silence radiating through the salty mist at high speed. Vijay had not just offered to give us a ride, but had given us the feeling of taking flight in the wide-open sea.

We turned slightly, making a wide arc, and I leaned a little to balance myself as the boat began to slow. We came to a near stop, the motor still rumbling, though its roaring scream had been silenced. Now the air moved around us, rather than us through it. In the relative stillness, the waves danced against the side of the boat and caused it to rock a little. It gave us the same cradling feeling we had used to calm the children in the villages. I looked over the edge to admire the near-indigo blue color of the water. In the distance, the shoreline appeared as though it could have been Venice Beach, for I had seen it many times from boat rides on Santa Monika Bay, but the deep alluring hues of this Bay of Bengal water elicited as many mysteries as the multitude of spectacles ashore.

Without a word, we looked at one another with an unrestrained expression of exhilaration, Mitta and I for the wonderful adventure, Vijay and the fishermen for their opportunity to share it with us. Vijay turned the boat toward shore and began to throttle the motor, building back more speed; the ride was back on. With the same enthrall, we made the return trip to shore. Along the way, we encountered another vessel, fishermen returning late. We passed with a nod and wave of recognition from Vijay and continued our trek to the beach.

Almost too quickly, we arrived near the breaking waves and Vijay slowed the craft. The waves were not so large that they would be any threat to the boat, but they did give us a bit of a push when we got in front of them. I continued my stance in the boat, wrapped in a Walter Mitty-esque daydream of conquest or discovery. The boat floated as though in slow motion onto the sand and I easily stepped over the side into the calf-high water. Dhamu and Mitta followed in like manner as we all, having gained our sea legs, struggled to walk unwaveringly on land.

As we approached a kattumaram sitting high on the beach, we observed several children sitting, as though waiting for our return. One of the children was the young girl we had treated in the previous clinic. She was dressed in attractive attire, as though she had come from school. She greeted Mitta like a beloved Auntie. The two walked together, hand in hand, back to the houses fronting the beach as Dhamu and I followed. Vijay and his companions completed their work securing the boat and motor.

As we were nearing a house on the beach, the young girl's mother, who also had received treatment, came out to greet us. She was also dressed in fine clothing and her hair had been curled. She excitedly told us that she had just returned from a day of work at the market, selling the fish the men had brought from the sea that morning. She showed us the rupees she had earned then invited us inside for a visit. We stepped into the tiny cinderblock home that, like the others, had only two small rooms. There was no furniture in either room and the second room had a large hole in the roof through which sunlight poured, accentuating its emptiness.

Seated on the floor in the front room was the woman's mother. She tended a small fire in a pot, atop which was a stew pot. Also adorned in finer clothing, she moved like a priestess at the altar, adding this ingredient and that ingredient to the pot, particularly small fish that had been lying on the floor beside her. We took our places on the floor, leaning against the wall on the far side of the room. Cold drinks were offered, accepted, served, and enjoyed.

"It is like a new day," the woman said. "We have waited to return to our work and now we feel as though our lives will continue to move forward."

Only days before she had worn a mask of despair; today her face radiated with hope. Together we celebrated their recovery and the signs that the other villagers may also gain the same hope. She thanked us for our help once more. Despite our happiness at the return of her emotional well-being, the open-sky view in the next room reminded us that recovery would come in stages, one mending project at a time.

We completed our visit and stepped out into the midday sun. Together, we all walked back to the main road where the motorbikes had been parked. Along the way the young girl walked firmly embracing Mitta, who held her like one who had been rescued from a great distress. Mitta would return to the states later that night, but she made a promise to return and continue to help the family, particularly to help repair the damaged roof of their home. As we left Srinivasapuram, the villagers stood waving as they, and the village, disappeared behind us.

Rather that turning right to return to town, we turned left to cross the bridge toward Adyar. Near the same area that we had purchased rice, we stopped at a small stall-like shop filled with sewing machines and accessories. The machines were unlike those that I had seen in the states, bearing greater resemblance to the classic machine my mother had used, or more closely to the professional machines with simple desks that my childhood friends, Bryon and Bennie Test, had in their upholstery shop. Dhamu and Vijay set to work describing the machine they were looking for, then agreed to a price and completed the sale. Contented that we had secured a good deal on a proper machine for the tailor and his family, we headed back to town.

There was still packing to be done at the hotel before a full evening of farewells. We had also been contacted by the Yoga instructor from the small hospital across from the hotel and learned that we could participate in a class at 5 pm. As we rode back to the hotel, Mitta continued to take in all the sites around, as though she could hold them in her heart and mind. When we arrived at the hotel, she asked to be dropped off at the street where, with her familiar greeting to the vendors, she purchased a final cup of tea.

24

Departure

The midwinter sun glimmered golden hues on the trees and buildings as it neared completion of this day's journey. Amidst the growing shadows on the hospital rooftop, we sat quietly, cross-legged, listening to the gentle instruction of Sri Latte. "In the West," she said, "death is considered to be a bad thing. One does all one can to avoid it, struggling with an angrily clenched fist and body, resisting the inevitable. In an effort to avoid death, they are pushing life away from them, rejecting their very breath and bringing themselves closer to death with each hesitant inhalation."

"In the East, we consider death to be our destination. From our birth, we are on a journey to our own death. Because of this consideration, we desire to have a good journey and arrive at our destination satisfied. We grasp the breath as it comes to us, make it a part of ourselves, and use it to help fulfill our great hope for fullness of life."

A birdsong rose from the trees below us, floating on the din of early evening traffic, punctuated with car horns and the rhythm of human activities.

"Many come to learn of this yoga practice, considering the stretching and contorting of the body into the familiar 'asanas' or postures. This is an important method to train and balance the body, but first we must learn the way of simply being, to receive each breathing moment of life, grasping it and making it our own. The force of life is in the breath. We call it "prana" and we call the practice of learning to use the breath "pranayama". This is where we will begin our practice. Perhaps we will not have the ability to obtain or hold the delicate asanas, but if we can effectively practice pranayama, the force of our lives will be with us always, whether in our special postures or in our everyday lives."

"Let us sit together in silence, no effort, only the breath."

During the next hour, Sri Latte guided us through many different methods of drawing breath through nostrils, through the mouth with teeth closed, through one nostril at a time. She taught us to hold the breath within, at different levels of the trunk, and how to disperse the gathered breath within. She taught us to create internal locks in the throat and how to intensify the breath within through rapid cycles that caused the body to warm as though we had fanned the fires of our being. Throughout these lessons I took pleasure in familiar and new techniques and understanding, but was most struck by the transformation in our guru. She had begun the instruction as a gentle and angelic guide, but as the exercises intensified, so did her own countenance. As I felt my own body warm and tingle with the electrifying oxygenation, I watched her body and face transform with nostrils flaring like that of a dragon breathing fire.

Following our pranayama practice, Sri Latte began to guide us through various stretches and postures I had known since my teens. These familiar forms in this new place transported me back to that time, reviewing the path this yoga practice would take me over decades, a thread connecting chapters of my life. With each motion and hesitation, I anchored again to the steady flow and distribution of the breath within.

In time, we found ourselves lying still on our backs, resting atop small carpets instead of the rubber mat familiar from our visits to Santa Monica's Yoga Works. In the stillness of our centers, with the orchestra of life continuing its movement about us, we began the ubiquitous progressive relaxation of the "corpse pose", though as we continued, a new adventure was added. "Imagine yourself as though you are a kite floating high in the sky, attached to a long string. Set yourself free. Dance upon the wind." With those words my mind took flight high above the hospital, the street, India, and all time.

I had first learned this progressive relaxation technique as a teen at the Oklahoma Summer Arts Institute. My mime teacher, Tony Montanaro, used the method to induce trance and guide us through visualization in order to carry our consciousness from our own form to that of an animal. This powerful "I AM" method liberated and empowered my character development and performance capabilities. For twenty years I used and taught this technique, cultivating a shortcut instant projection skill that transformed both my improvisational abilities and sense of social interconnectedness.

In 1995 I learned a self-hypnosis method from Gil Boyne that also included the progressive relaxation. Days after learning the technique, Lenise and I took a weekend camping trip to Joshua Tree Park. Eager to practice my new skill in a favorite environment, I climbed high on one of the massive granite-quartz mounds of Jumbo Rocks Campground. With me, I carried a small kite.

Once upon my perch, I launched the kite into the forceful desert breeze and let out the string until it danced high above me. I lay down on my back, kite string in hand, half-closed my eyes, and with each exhalation, released my mind from my body to take flight as the kite. Freedom, exhilaration, and boundless choreography beyond my crystallized childhood dream as dancer Rudolph Nureyev brought rapture to the marrow of my soul. My experience came to inform my therapeutic work, as I would later tailor the "I AM" as an expansive healing exercise.

Now, one decade later, I was given the similar flight on the far side of the earth. Time, space, and infinite possibility embraced and uplifted me again. I would have been content to stay in this place until cold or craving brought me back to my physical existence. Sri Latte, with her skill, guided us back gently, as though it was our choice and the timely thing to do. After a few moments of quiet observation, we rolled up our carpets and gave them to Sri Latte. Thanking her for her fine instruction, we placed hands together and said "Vanakam, Nanthree."

The light of day had almost vanished when we returned to the hotel to prepare for Mitta's departure. We still had some time before Dhamu's scheduled arrival to take us for dinner at his family's home, so we decided to take a stroll for her to say farewell to the elegant little white temple around the corner. As we approached, we noticed a stir of activity, unlike our previous visit. The lights were on and though we did not enter, we could see through the protective grating surrounding the open court that a priest and his student sat together reviewing their own lessons. We did not want to disturb them, so, contented with our visit, we turned to walk away. As we were admiring the carved figures adorning the top of the temple, we heard a voice speaking English behind us.

"Greetings, where are you traveling from?" The voice inquired.

I turned to see a man standing nearby. "We are from the U.S. We have come to help with tsunami recovery." I answered.

"Thank you for your efforts, I'm sure you are making a difference for some people who have suffered greatly." He looked up at the figures we had been admiring. "It must seem strange to you. Most westerners who visit think that this Hindu religion is quite foreign. All these deities can cause one to wonder, but at its core, Hinduism is a monotheistic religion. There is really only one great God. All of these others are merely his helpers, like saints, if you will."

Having been raised Catholic and taught the veneration of the Saints at the church and in my grandmother's garden and home, I suddenly understood the panoply of the different aspects of life that each of these Hindu deities fulfilled in individuals' lives. Such was the patron of all comings and goings, Ganesha or "Ganapati", the elephant-headed god whose image was on every corner, every shop, every home, and every vehicle. He had been a favorite "saint" for both Lenise and me for decades. As "the remover of obstacles", his image had given strength through our varied endeavors and adventures.

"Even the great trinity" he continued, "is simply three forms of the same great God. Vishnu, the sustainer, is always depicted reclining, for his work is done. Brahma, the creator rises from the navel of the dreaming Vishnu to craft the material world. Shiva, the destroyer, is the third of this great trinity. Through his reduction of all that has been made manifest, he provides for the continuing cycle of regeneration. These three gods or forces in harmony are what keep the world churning.

In fact, the carved images that are seen in the temples are only representations of the God who lives inside. If you see people praying in the temple, you will see them looking down or closing their eyes. The priest is in the small shrine circling the flaming lamp around the deity, but the devotee does not look on. Instead, his eyes are closed so that he can embrace the image of this god within him."

I recalled this behavior from our temple visits and now it made perfect sense to me. What appeared to be the reverence that I had learned growing up to "not look upon the face of God," was indeed the effort to see or know the presence of God within. Suddenly, this religion did not seem foreign at all. Just as the crucifix was not a "graven image", neither were these idols. They were only symbols of something much more intangible than what could be fashioned through wood or stone.

"I have a gift for you," the gentleman said before dashing around the corner. He returned with a small paperback book that he placed in my hand. "This should give you information for continued study, as I can tell that you are one who seeks greater knowledge." I looked down at the title of the small volume and read "The Symbolism of Hindu Gods and Rituals". It was exactly my kind of book!

"Thank you very much," I said. "You have opened a world of understanding to me. I will treasure this knowledge you have shared."

"You are most welcome," he responded, "share this knowledge with others and return again to visit our wonderful mother India. And thank you again for the help that you have brought to the people."

With that we all bowed "Vanakam Nanthree" then returned to the hotel to gather Mitta's bags and meet Dhamodharan.

Basker pulled the autorickshaw up to the covered entrance of the Ram Guest House and he, Vijay, and Dhamu climbed out to greet us. They loaded the stack of Mitta's bags and together we all pressed ourselves back into the auto and rolled down the quiet drive.

Dhamu's home was now familiar to us as we disembarked from the auto and walked down the outdoor corridor to the front door. We entered a celebratory, though somewhat sad gathering. Dhamu's mother invited us to the back bedroom to make prayers before their household altar. She waved hands of blessing over us and anointed us with the familiar yellow and red clay powder. There was a stirring about

Mitta and both Dhamu's mother and sisters expressed their care and sadness at her approaching departure.

We returned to the front room where mats were placed for another delicious meal. Dhamu's sisters brought out channa masala, chapatti, and cold drinks. We received the food with gratitude and savored each bite, commenting on the special care that had been given for Mitta's final meal in India. We ate beyond our needs as ladle after ladle of delicious food was delivered to our plates. Contentedly overfilled, we sat back to rest and enjoy the remaining time with the family.

Dhamu's nephew, Deepash, stepped forward with a small yellow plastic box and sat before Mitta. With arms reaching out to deliver the package, he looked into Mitta's eyes and said, "My gift to you." She opened the box to reveal a wide assortment of bangles and stickers and hair ornaments. She lifted each tiny treasure from the box and admired it with a sense of wonder, not so much about the item, but with the tenderness with which it was delivered.

Each of the sisters brought forward similar packages and presented them in the same way, holding the item, looking squarely into Mitta's eyes, and expressing "My gift to you." The pile of treasures was building before her when Dhamu stepped forward with a large package.

"On that first night after the tsunami, as we huddled shivering on the sidewalk, all our possessions stolen by the sea, a kind stranger gave us this blanket. It was our only protection from the cold of the night." He produced a simple woven blanket from the bag. "We would like for you to take this blanket to Jim Uncle, to give him a token of how his help has protected us from further suffering. There are two other blankets here that we also received at that time. We make these blankets a gift to each of you, so you may also remember that we are so thankful for the care that you have brought to our family, our village, and the people of India."

The blankets were thin but carried the weight of suffering and hope. We accepted them as one would a sacrament, with humble respect. Mitta found room in her tightly packed bag for her blanket while I gathered mine and Jim Uncle's to pack with my things.

Outside, the dusk of early evening had progressed to darkness and the time for farewell arrived. Mitta embraced each of the family members with tears and the team climbed back into the auto and drove off toward the airport.

The drive seemed longer in the autorickshaw, but its openness allowed us to experience a greater sense of the now-familiar city. In time, we arrived at the airport and parked at the opposite end of the terminal than where we had arrived. As we loaded her luggage cart, Mitta spent time saying goodbye to the guys, giving each a special speech about their time together and her counsel for their continued growth. In these expanded minutes, she appeared as Dorothy saying her farewells to the Scarecrow, Tin Man, and Lion before departing Oz.

We said goodbye amid discussion of details of the continued work in India and tasks for Mitta to address when she returned to the States. Our business complete, she grasped the handles of the luggage cart, as much her guide as her aid, and rolled forward to join the line of passengers awaiting security screening. We all stood watching as she passed through the doors with one last wave goodbye.

Together, we climbed back into the now roomier auto and began the silent drive back to the hotel.

25

Scouting

I crept out of bed at 6:30 a.m. and stumbled across the street to attend yoga class. The light was stirring, but the sun had not yet fully risen. I was excited by the prospect of having said goodbye and hello to the sun from the same spot. I climbed the four flights of stairs to the rooftop and took my place with the two other students there for the early morning session. I rolled out the small piece of carpet, sat, stretched a little, and spent time in meditation before the session began.

Sri Latte guided us patiently through our pranayama and asanas. The gray light of early morning turned golden as we flowed through our poses. By the time we had finished, the morning sun was reaching down to press upon us with piercing heat.

I had brought my flute with me, and upon completion of the session, I told Sri Latte that I had come prepared to share a song. She invited me to play for the group. We all remained on our carpet pads as I played out a song of morning and gratitude for my new instructor and the privilege of studying yoga in its homeland. When I finished playing, they all expressed gratitude for the song and curiosity for the strange Native American flute.

As the other students and I were rolling our carpets, Sri Latte approached me. "I have always wanted to learn to play the flute," she said. "I even had a teacher for awhile, but he lost patience with me. Do you think you could teach me a little? We could even trade lessons. I will teach you yoga and you can teach me to play the flute."

"I would be happy to," I said. "We can even begin right now if you would like." I looked around on the roof and saw that the small eastern wall was casting a shadow on the rooftop. "Come, let's sit here in the shade so we can be comfortable."

We sat together facing one another. I held the flute in my hand with all of the holes open and brought it toward my face. "First, we just learn to blow through the flute itself." I brought the flute to my lips and blew a long steady note. Then, using a cloth to wipe the mouthpiece, passed the flute to Sri Latte. She took the flute in her hands, carefully mimicking the same manner of holding as I had used, then brought the flute to her lips and let a timid note rise from the flute. Her eyes looked up at mine as she inhaled and blew again with confidence. A nice, sustained note flowed from the flute.

"This is much easier," she said, still holding and examining the flute. "The other flute I tried to play had a different kind of mouthpiece. I had to blow across a hole and hold it out to the side. It was very difficult." She placed the flute against her lips and blew again, smiling and looking at it as she withdrew it. "Yes, this is much easier to play."

I took the flute, held it with all holes closed and brought it to my lips to blow out a low tone. I then lifted one finger at a time to produce a progression of notes. I played up and down the scale, then passed the flute to her to allow her to do the same. She diligently covered each hole with a finger then brought it to her mouth to blow another, now much lower tone. She looked up at me with pleasure and began lifting each finger in the same manner.

The Native American flute has a peculiar fingering technique. It is designed with only six holes on the top that are covered with the first three fingers of each hand, similar to an Irish pennywhistle. However, in simple scale playing of the flute, the third finger hole from the top is kept covered. This is a bit strange at first, but one becomes accustomed to it in time. Many flute sellers will wrap a strap of leather around the hole to keep it covered for the novice player.

I took care to demonstrate this method as I showed Sri Latte the scale technique. She played up the scale and then back down, just as I had demonstrated. Her eyes and smile brightened as she held the flute forward looking at it, saying "this flute is much easier to play, I can actually make several notes that sound almost like a song. I could never do this with my other flute lesson." She held the flute close and played a few more scales, changing out the notes, listening for a tune.

"You are an excellent student of the flute," I said.

"Because you are an excellent flute guru," she replied.

"I think that is enough for today," I said, "we can learn a little more when I come for another class. For you to truly learn, you will need a flute. I will begin searching for one for you."

With that, our lessons were complete for the day. We departed the rooftop together as the sun was chasing the last shadows away. I crossed the street and returned to my room to prepare for a full day out with Dhamodaran.

Since Mitta had departed, we considered relocating to simpler accommodations nearer Dhamu's home. I hopped on the back of the two-wheeler and we set out on our adventure. Our first stop was at an increasingly familiar area, the Kapaleeswarar Temple in Mylapore. This is the majestic temple area I had first been enchanted by while on a late evening ride with Dhamu. It had been Friday night and the temple was very active. At the time it seemed a great mystery to turn down a dusty road and emerge before a spectacular brightly-colored and gilded structure, highly illuminated and teeming with activity. It was at this same temple bazaar area that we had shopped in with Mitta.

The area was much more subdued during mid-day. On a street facing the temple complex, Dhamu parked the bike and we both dismounted. "Here Uncle, let us first see if there is a room here for you." We climbed a narrow, dim flight of stairs to a small office where a clerk greeted us and spoke energetically with Dhamu.

"This would be a good place, but there is no room for you here now, let us continue our search." We descended the stairs and returned to the plaza.

Once on the street, I noticed an eyeglass shop on the adjacent corner. I had received an eye exam shortly before leaving L.A., but did not have time to get the new prescription filled. I had already seen eyeglass shops at different locations and browsed for styles. This shop looked inviting, and after searching for a few minutes, I found a nice pair of wire frames that seemed my style. I tried them on and Dhamu agreed it was a "smart" look for me. I produced my prescription from my wallet and gave it to the clerk. He told me the glasses would be ready in two days; the price for frames and lenses, about sixteen US dollars.

Dhamu had located a nice "American Hotel" restaurant with AC, so we stepped inside and had a quick lunch of rice and channa masala. We motored away from the temple district and headed toward Dhamu's neighborhood. On the way, he stopped to offer me a special treat. We entered a small music shop, not unlike in any city. It had a small entry area with a counter that had a variety of instruments on display. Through a passageway lay another larger room with even more exotic yet familiar instruments. We approached the counter and inquired about flutes.

The clerk showed us several different instruments, mostly similar to the narasthwara I had purchased in Pondicherry. They were of varying sizes, like those we had heard at the wedding celebration. He showed us a lovely transverse-styled flute as well. The instrument I desired the most was a wooden version of the cast one I had already acquired. Its price was above my meager budget, but I did purchase an extra supply of the finely crafted double reeds. There was no simple flute that I could take for Sri Latte; so, after thanking the clerk, we departed.

Back on the two-wheeler, we left a dusty trail en route to our next destination. Jim Uncle had suggested that we look at rooms at the modest compound where he stayed while in town. It was farther south, even past Srinivasapuram, near the Theosophical Society in Adyar. The buildings, a pale terracotta color, arose as though formed from the dusty soil they rested upon. We rounded a corner and there, in stark contrast, stood a mighty banyan tree. Its grey and green, juxtaposed against the dusty ground and buildings, gave it an even mightier presence. This tree reminded me of a similar Banyan tree in a park in Beverly Hills in whose branches I have spent much time resting. Again, I felt connected to this far away place.

We strolled through the complex of small buildings until, at last, finding the office. We were shown a couple of very simple rooms, with AC and without. Though these rooms seemed quite sufficient for one on a hermitage, we concluded that the comfort of Ram Guest House was also a good value and would do nicely for my remaining days in India. It was reassuring to know, however, that when I returned to India one day, I already had a familiar and comforting place to stay.

26

Of Many, One

Dhamu motored across town to a site he wanted me to see. We arrived at a large, nearly empty, plaza. Railings divided the space, like 'people-mover' lines at an amusement park. We approached a building that appeared to be a Christian church, having a great cross-crowned spire rising from its center, but it was like no cathedral or church building I had seen. Its architecture seemed more byzantine or old-world, with a brown and white checked façade pitching out to small square towers on the corners.

As we drew nearer, I noticed a steel-grate barricade around a giant niche beside the courtyard. This I readily recognized as a shrine of some type, and as I approached, my guess was confirmed by the presence of many small pieces of string tied around small pieces of wood and attached to the grating. These were clearly prayer offerings left by supplicants. I was reminded of the small room outside the sacred hole of dirt at the Santuario de Chimayo in New Mexico. As a child I visited this site with my family and stood awestruck at the walls hung with row after row of crutches and braces left behind by those whose faith had set them free of their need. They looked like the tack on the wall in my grandfather's barn, but rather than bridles and reins meant to restrain, these artifacts testified to a need that had been released. It was, in part, these walls in the Santuario, and the healing power of faith to which they gave witness, that inspired me to pursue a life in the healing arts.

Here in this place, I also connected with the needs of those who had left their emblems of hope tethered to the point of promise. Within the grating stood a great tree, constructed of concrete, whose branches reached out to form the ceiling and walls of the small shrine. Within the branches of the tree was a statue of Mary holding the infant Jesus, the "Madonna and Child". At the feet, statues of individuals making offerings suggested to me that the site commemorated a visitation of the "Mother of God" near this place.

Dhamu guided me within the church itself. It was unlike any church I had visited in the United States or Europe, except perhaps the Russian Orthodox Church in Geneva, with its gilded icons. Here were similar images encased in glass and surrounded by ornate metal. In stark contrast to anything I had seen before, however, was the uniquely Indian flair of small golden dots of powder applied at various points, including many finger marks at the feet of the image. Joining tradition, I kissed my fingers and touched the feet of the image to show my respect.

We walked from the small anti-room into the great pavilion of the church, and then strolled back out into the plaza. A small dirt street extended down to the right of the church, fronting the beach. Many souvenir stalls lined the street. Near the stalls sat a woman with many carved block stamps laid out on a blanket. Together, we searched through them, Dhamu demonstrating their value by having the woman press the block on a red pad, then stamping the image onto his palm. I searched through all of the various designs, finding a small perched bird that seemed a perfect gift for Lenise.

Still embraced by the far-reaching impact of the Virgin in the shrine, I decided that I should commemorate this place by acquiring rosaries for my Catholic nieces. We perused several stalls until finding just the right items at the right price. "Now," I turned to tell Dhamu, "they must be blessed by the priest." Together, we pivoted to return to the church.

A small door at the side of the inner pavilion seemed to be a staff office. We approached the office and asked if a priest was available to bless the rosaries. We were told that he had gone to lunch and we should wait one hour for his return, but within a few minutes, a young priest emerged from the office and walked to the middle of the pavilion to greet us.

I held up the treasured trinkets with a measure of meekness. "They are for my nieces," I said. "They are very precious to me and I would like to carry a blessing of this place to them." My voice broke, I felt a swelling knot in my throat, and the room began to blur as tears rushed into my eyes. The priest reached out in that way it seems only priests do, and taking my trembling hand, withdrew a small vial of holy water and placed a little on each. Passing his hands over the rosaries, he began to pray.

I closed my eyes to receive the prayer blessing and felt the room open around me. There had been other visitors milling about and the sounds of their presence remained with me as I drifted out beyond this place and time. My grandmother's presence was beside me, silently expressing gratitude for my faithfulness in this place, for remembering to give respect to Mary and the saints, for remembering the gentle lessons she had shown me as a small child, and for following my heart to convey this same caring to those beloved young ladies and all my nieces and nephews who mean so much to me and her. I don't know how long the prayer continued. I am sure it was brief, but the reverberating sense of spirit and love felt like an embrace of eternity. I opened my eyes. The room and the others were still there as they had been. The light was still the same, but the priest looked directly at me, knowingly, and with a little gratitude himself.

We exited the church again into the bright sun. This time I felt quite different, as though an important task had been completed and thus I was more fulfilled. We strolled back down the dusty street, greeting the vendors as we did. A group of small boys, about three to five years old, approached us. We shook hands and offered to take their photo, an entertaining treat from visitors. We strolled on until reaching a simple but substantial temple at the end of the road, a bookend to the church at the other end.

"Uncle, this temple is closed now, so we cannot go inside, but it is a very special temple. It is for Lakshmi, the great goddess."

I thought it intriguing that this Lakshmi temple would be here where the church so apparently sacred to Mary stood. This place also seemed to have the presence of the "Great Mother". I stood still, looking at the temple, seeking again to feel that motherly spirit.

As we were walking away, I noticed a woman sitting near the front of the temple. She was begging for rupees and held up her hand as I walked past. I reached into my pocket to produce a few rupees for her and as I handed them to her I noticed that her lower right leg was very swollen and dark. I placed hands together, not in honor, but in supplication, then looked and gestured at her leg, seeking permission to give her treatment. She looked at her leg and then back to me, as if to confirm her discomfiting despair. I turned my palms toward the leg, and still holding them a couple of feet away, began to move my hands slightly toward the leg, as if to convey that I was sending healing to her.

To my surprise, she shrank a little away from me, quickly grabbed her blue chiffon-like scarf and pulled it over her face, and began to make prayer like gestures. I continued giving her the Reiki treatment, and she patiently indulged my efforts. I remembered the scholar we had met at the temple telling me that it was tradition to look away from the god. In my bewildered mind, I thought to myself, "That's strange; she is behaving toward me as though I am a god." I received it as respect, in that Reiki is not from me, but simply my effort to support one's divine healing potential.

We walked to the open beach and trod along the sand back to where the motorbike was parked. From the beach perspective, the church and the temple, connected by the street of shops, appeared as one single complex, reinforcing my sense that though there were two disparate religions represented here, they were unified in one single ideal, the love of the Mother.

There was still one stop on our day's journey. Jim Uncle had recommended that, if possible, we visit the Theosophical Society headquarters in Adyar. We had passed its entrance several times on our journeys south, so I was pleased to finally pass through the gates and learn more about a tradition I had been vaguely familiar with for decades. We stopped by the visitors' center then strolled through the grounds.

We came upon a simple, yet majestic building. The façade had white columns and red panels, the center of which bore a near life-sized relief of an elephant head. We walked inside and I was instantly taken by its elegant simplicity. Many reliefs of religious figures adorned the walls and inscribed over the top of a great entryway were the words "There is no religion higher than truth". I was meditating on the words when I heard a strange voice behind me say "Welcome."

Dhamu and I turned to see a graceful woman in her seventies with white hair and western dress. At first I thought her accent English, but I learned soon it was Australian. I think she said her name was Helen. She invited us into a small room off the foyer we were standing near. We sat together and talked. We talked of our work in India: the honor with which we had been received by the villagers; the privilege we felt of being invited into their lives; the remarkable strength and resilience they had demonstrated; the genuine kindness and gratitude they had expressed to us. We spoke of the history of the project with the Center, of Jim Uncle's time spent there over so many years and the bridge that was built through his relationship with Narayanan, Dhamu's father.

She told us of the many years during which she and her husband had traveled there for summer retreats, and how they had finally determined that here, on these grounds, in the heart of coastal South India, was where they wanted to spend all of their time, and had come here as permanent residents. Time passed like a breeze, gentle and refreshing on a warm day. We thanked each other for our delight at meeting at this time during each of our journeys and departed, with her recommendation, to stroll through the grounds.

We walked by many small buildings, like dormitories, observing the quiet comings and goings of individuals. We observed the many varieties of trees that were growing, and the many flowers on trees, shrubs, and in the beds themselves. It was like vast botanical gardens. Following the paved path, we arrived at a crossroads where we met an old Indian man wearing a white lungi folded short, a whitish shirt, and a white turban. He was holding a staff of bamboo, about his height. He motioned me to walk one direction at the crossroads, as though the other one had been closed. We followed his instruction and continued on the open road.

As we walked, Dhamu turned toward me. "Uncle, I would like to make a suggestion. I think we should offer this man some rupees. See, he is old; he has many people whom he is taking care of. Let us offer him some rupees for tea."

I turned back toward the man and approached him, offering him some rupees while making the familiar gesture for tea. A pleasant smile of surprise lit up his face. He took the money and gave thanks with hands together. I offered a salute in return.

He turned and gestured to a sign that was near him. It was down the path that had been closed, so I looked at him for consent to go down the path. He nodded and waved us forward. As I walked toward the sign I noticed the grove of delicate trees that lined the pathway. As I followed them upward, I saw that they were all connected to great branches, all joined together. I had known of the great banyan tree, whose branches send great shoots to the ground to become as trees themselves, but for the first time I was in the place of a great banyan "forest". Even the grand banyan I had spent so many hours nestled in the branches of in Beverly Hills had only a few tendrils dancing toward the ground, and none as developed as these.

There is a splendid silence one can find when pausing in the middle of a stand of woods. I stood and felt myself in the brotherhood of the slender wooden friends. I felt their connection to each other, all part of the same organism. I followed the branches to the mighty trunk, from which I could almost take in the scale of the entire tree. Near the trunk, beside the trail, was the sign. We walked forward and read:

> "This banyan tree, whose hospitality you are enjoying, is one of the largest in the world. From north to south it measures 238ft. From east to west 250 ft. The total area exceeds 59, 500 sq ft. It is a unique specimen. Two others, equally large, are known to exist, but one of them the central trunk has rotted away, and

the other appears to have originally consisted of two trees which have since grown together.

This tree continues to grow, and from the mother root extend many offspring.

It has been the centre of many notable gatherings of the Theosophical Society and thousands of visitors have rested in its shade."

I knew of the banyan tree, the bodhi tree that the Buddha had sat under. I considered that to have spent much time isolated in the quintessence of such a grand being as this tree, I could both lose and find myself over and over again.

My reverie was interrupted by the "guard" waving his stick toward us and pointing down the pathway. We turned to look and saw a large white Brahma bull pulling a cart toward us. He bore a yoke of wood, but the poles that were attached connected to a flatbed cart with modern rubber wheels. Another old gentleman was piloting the cart, which was piled high with cuttings of plant material. A younger man walked beside the cart to help navigate it through the narrow path. We greeted the old man, who invited us to sit with him for photos.

We strolled a little ahead of the cart, then said our goodbye and headed toward the gates. Our visit was drawing to a close as the afternoon sun began casting long shadows, signaling the finish of the day. We stopped at the bookstore on the way out. I purchased some incense and pocket volumes of the three great teachings of Theosophy: *The Voice of the Silence, At the Feet of the Master,* and *Light on the Path.* I found a copy of *The Science of Yoga* by Patanjali that I really wanted, but refused the purchase for consideration of cost and carry.

We rolled out of the gates of calm, back onto the busied and noisy roadways of Chennai.

27

Guy Time

We arrived in Srinivasapuram as the sun was drifting low in the sky, casting golden hues on all it illuminated. There was a commotion on the beach near our tarp-covered treatment "clinic". Several children surrounded a group parading from the beach to the village proper. We approached and met the entourage near the ruins of Vijay's house. The children parted to reveal a middle-aged man carrying a small bag. When they realized I was there, a chant began to arise from the group, compelling the man carrying the bag to reveal his treasure to me. He set the bag on the ground and opened it for me to clearly see what appeared like sand-covered ping-pong balls. I quickly realized they were turtle eggs.

He reached into the bag and produced one of the eggs, holding it forth for me to examine it. A glint of pride sparkled in his eye, satisfaction at his successful find. The clamor arose from the children again as the man carefully peeled the egg, revealing a brilliant yellow yolk beneath the soft, thin white shell. He held out the naked egg in the palm of his hand for me to see clearly. The clamor rose higher. He brought his hand to his mouth and in a single sea-bird like gesture, gulped the egg, leaned his head back, and let the treat roll down his throat with an enthusiastic swallow. He looked back at me with a grin, seeking to read my own delight and surprise.

I remembered the roofer in the small Oklahoma town that I spent much of my childhood in teaching me how to suck eggs at age eleven. Like many of the children present at this demonstration, I had watched with squeamish wonder as he pierced holes in top and bottom of the egg, then placed lips on the larger hole and sucked out the egg, passing the emptied shell on to me for investigation. I found the trick to be easy and the brief rich slimy flavor of the egg soon passed into self-satisfaction. I was happy to see that like so many things, our lives followed similar developmental tracks. I applauded the man for his brave stunt and celebrated his good fortune with him for his cache.

He gathered up the bag and the celebrants around him and continued his parade. Dhamu and I followed close behind, not because we wanted to continue the party, but because there was an important visit for us to make in the village.

We strolled down the now-familiar village road, greeting the neighbors at their posts as we did. A group of young children approached us singing a song. Dhamu stopped to show me that several of them wore matching clothing. "Here, Uncle, are the school uniforms we have provided for the children with help from Jim Uncle and others." There were both blue and green shorts and skirts with matching checkered shirts. The children looked sharp and proud in their uniforms and I understood Dhamu's mission to help provide them.

We continued down the road to a small house. On the wall beside the door, a tic-tac-toe had been scratched into the plaster, played out, and a second chart with numbers had been drawn next to it, emblems of the immediacy of childhood play. Dhamu knocked on the door and we were invited inside. Here was the woman we had spent time giving care to earlier, though transformed from her demeanor of sorrow to one of happiness.

She escorted us to the tiny back room occupied by her tailor husband and a brand-new sewing machine with table. It was the equipment we had purchased to help this family continue its recovery from the loss of their daughter and livelihood. They showed us their gratitude for the gift with many expressions of "Nanthree". They then posed for a photo with their two children beside the machine. The bright glow in their faces brought great warmth to my heart.

We exited back on to the street, trailed by a growing pack of children. A fellow about the same age as Dhamodharan approached and began speaking with him. He pointed my direction and they both looked at me, then continued conversing. Dhamu walked toward me. "Uncle," he said, "this good friend has heard of some of the help you have been able to give others. He is asking if he can have some time to receive help from you now."

"Of course," I said, and we continued our stroll back to the small canopy at the beach, this time escorted by one in need.

We arrived at the small shelter and the three of us sat together in the sand. Dhamu spoke with him briefly and turned toward me. "Uncle, this man is a fisherman. He works very hard in a very difficult situation. All day, from before the sun, he is fighting and fighting. He fights the sea, he fights the nets, and he fights the fish. This fighting is making his body very tight, like stone, and this tightness is causing much pain. Many fishermen find relief from this pain at the wine shop, but this only makes the problem worse. He is concerned that the sea will win, that this tightness in his body will break him and he will be unable to continue his work. Is there some First Medicines treatment that can help him?"

"Yes," I said, "first we must teach his body to be less tight, we must help him to relax his muscles and calm his mind. When he knows that he can be free of this tightness and pain, he will know that he can continue to work and have his life. Let's give him treatment now."

TSUNAMI EFFECT

Dhamu instructed the man to lie down on the mat beside us and gained his permission for touch. I felt along the sides of his legs and realized his tension had become fixed in his muscles, causing them to be as dense as stone. It seemed as though the salt of the sea had drawn the very water from his sinews, leaving only constricted flesh behind.

I placed one hand on his forehead and instructed him to focus on his breathing. "Each time you exhale," I said, "you naturally relax. Each time you exhale now, allow yourself to naturally relax more and more." I listened as Dhamu translated and watched his body begin to limply surrender to the soft sand beneath him. I lifted one hand and let the arm hang in space, encouraging him to let it swing freely like the branch of a tree then swayed the hand to and fro to help the arm and shoulder relax more. Once observing the muscles slacken, I rested the hand upon his abdomen and encouraged him to let this relaxation flow to the rest of his body. I lifted his other hand and began to sway the arm in the same manner.

I continued guiding him through relaxation, asking him to tense the face muscles and then relax them. I guided him to allow the relaxation to flow from his face to neck and shoulders, compounding the calm I had already induced. I called out all of the sounds around us, the surf, the birds, and the sounds of the children playing. "Each of these familiar sounds can now give you calm and strength." I continued guiding him through each area of his body, calling out the same quality of comfortable relaxation as I did. I turned to Dhamu to ask for a report from our friend.

"So peaceful, I am so calm and relaxed." Dhamu translated his passive muttering.

"Know that it is you who are able to produce this good feeling," I said. "You can imagine yourself now at sea, still in command of the

184

tightness and calmness of your body. Feel your strength in arms and legs, feel your ability to be comfortable at all times, know the control that you possess."

Dhamu continued translating my instruction, then turned to me. "I have explained to him about his strongbody, Uncle."

After some time of rest, we brought him back to a wakeful state. He sat upright slowly, grinning at us as he did. He looked down at his hands, opening and closing them. He looked back at us with smiling eyes and said "Nanthree." He looked around at those on the beach as though he was seeing them in a different way than before. Together we rose and walked down toward the rolling waves.

The sun had now surrendered to the approaching night and descended beyond the horizon, taking the day's shadows with it and leaving only the evening gray behind. Villagers strolled along the waterfront as the cool air arrived at the beach.

We had filled the day with many adventures and now turned back toward the two-wheeler to return to the hotel and call the day complete.

28

Au Revoir Muttukadu

What had begun as weeks in India, remained now as only days. It was time to begin to say goodbye, to this ancient land of mystery, to this region filled with such history, to these people who were the living expression of both. I had come to give, to offer what tools I had to help allay the suffering of so many from such a globally unifying disaster. I had received treasured gifts that were illuminating how grand and gracious my world could be.

Dhamu met me at the hotel at mid-morning for our final trip to Muttukadu. With both glee and dread, I climbed aboard the back of the two-wheeler and our journey was under way. We traveled the same familiar route out of the city, the shops seeming so much closer and accessible from the bike. When we reached the open highway, I felt like a bullet fired from a gun, flying through open space with the wind against my face and my hair flowing freely. I braced against Dhamu as we sped forward, finally passing MGM and the road to the abandoned village. We arrived at the camp and dismounted the bike, stretching a little and looking about the encampment, which now seemed like the home of a kinsman.

We began to walk across the open field between the road and the tents as a young girl near the tents spied us and walked out to greet us. About five years old, she approached with the confidence and reassuring presence of an ambassador. She took my hand, as though she had been on watch for us, and escorted us into the camp. We navigated the tent ropes and passageways with steadying comments of guidance from our liaison, eventually arriving at her family's tent. Her parents greeted us and sent another villager to find Ramalinga. A place was provided for us to rest beneath a canopy outside an adjacent tent. Our young guide sat beside us with a calm sense of accomplishment.

I looked down at her with appreciation and she radiated back such a strong personal command that I felt I was in the graces of a young great soul. I had been impressed, since our arrival, at the remarkable beauty and power of the Tamil women, particularly those I met in the villages. Though living in marginal conditions near the sandy beach, and in some cases under tarp tents, I was struck by their ability to always appear as though they were dressed for an evening out, colorfully wrapped in vibrant sari and adorned with modest jewelry. Beyond their remarkable facial structure and rich dark skin, there was a spirit about these women, a strength that seemed to flow as though thru generations. This enduring nature could be observed in the school teachers, the young women and mothers of the infants, and most remarkably in the older women, the grandmothers. It was this manner that I observed in this young caretaker who had fearlessly brought us into her world. It was this and more.

I turned to her father, who was sitting with us. "Your daughter," I said, "is a very special person. She is brave and gentle and I see in her the mark of greatness. She will do mighty things in her life, and bring pride to both you and her village." He thanked me for my encouraging comments, and as Ramalinga arrived and sat with us, the girl rose and departed with her father to the adjacent tent.

"I want to thank you," I said to Ramalinga, "for allowing us to come and do our work with the people of your village. You have been like a friend, a brother, an 'uncle' indeed. It is time to return to my home. I will miss you and the friends I have come to know here in Muttukadu.

I will think of you often, and when I do, my heart will always be filled with happiness."

As Dhamu translated my remarks, I watched Ramalinga's head rocking left and right, the Tamil nod of acceptance. His face brightened as the report continued and he looked directly at me with compassionate, yet commanding eyes and said. "You have been like a gift sent in a very troubling time, bringing tools of comfort for the people and a spirit of kindness that will always be remembered. I thank you for this kindness that has brought you across this great distance. Please think of us and our appreciation for your help and come see us again when we have rebuilt our homes and returned to our village."

We sat a few moments longer, just enjoying being together. My young friend returned after a bucket bath at her tent with freshly washed hair and now wearing a red dress that in some ways matched the red and black batik shirt that I was wearing. We rose from our seats and as I picked up my backpack, she insisted on carrying it herself. Almost the same size as her, she could not raise it by its handle high enough to carry. By putting the shoulder straps on her shoulders, it could easily be carried on her back, though she now appeared as a little red beetle with a large shell. She reached up to take my hand and we continued our trek through camp.

Where I had previously observed wooden frames and some completed huts, now almost half of the tents had been transformed into row after row of small thatched huts. We walked through the several rows of huts until arriving at the home of Monika and her family. Happy to see us, her parents took us around the corner to find Monika and her sister playing. She looked up to see us and rose to give me a welcoming embrace. I squatted down to receive her hug and when I withdrew, she looked straight into my face and with slow, deliberate grace, closed and opened her previously paralyzed eyelid, slightly smiling with pride as she did. I let out a yelp and gave her an even more robust embrace.

Her parents joined into our celebration and told us that she had been receiving regular treatments at the hospital and they had been continuing her hands-on treatments at home. I gave her a brief treatment and, upon Dhamu's suggestion, gave some rupees to help with transportation for her treatments. Our parade continued.

Further down the row of huts, we were greeted by the father of the young troubled boy. He told us that his son was now at the school with the other children. He had stopped throwing stones and was not as distressed as before, but he had not yet begun to speak again, had not yet fully recovered. "Your love is helping him to heal," I said with encouragement. "Continue to help him as you have and he will continue to grow stronger each day." He thanked us for our help and with bows of "nanthree" we continued on.

Being early afternoon, school was still in session. Ramalinga led us down the path that led from the camp to the improvised school building. The teachers were glad to see us again and invited us inside the small building to speak with the students, all seated on the floor.

I entered the classroom and stood before the teacher's desk. "It is time for me to return to my home," I told the group of sixty or so young students. "I would like to leave you with a song, though; it is a song that you can remember in future times and recall the strangers who came from America to help you. At any time that you are sad, I want you to remember this song, a happy song, and remember that we are always thinking of you getting stronger...and smarter every day." The children laughed at Dhamu's translation and I put the flute to my lips and played out a song of gratitude, of sadness for loss, and of bright skipping happiness that comes after the sadness has been taken away.

When I finished the song I turned to thank the teachers; they offered their thanks also. As we stepped out of the classroom, the children were dismissed from school. They flowed out behind us into the open space between the two small buildings. They crowded around us and began to offer handshakes of thanks and farewell. Soon, what had begun as a group became a throng, each reaching out to shake hands and say "thanks." I reached out for every hand that I could, the group pressing and flowing around me, carrying us out of the courtyard and into the open field. I felt as though I was being borne up like a champion after a winning bout. We paused to take some photos then sadly, though buoyed with glee, turned toward the motorbike waiting by the road.

Our small entourage arrived at the two-wheeler, my young assistant still nobly toting my pack on her small back. We gathered together, embracing one another and taking photos, as though lingering would make the moment last forever. Reluctantly, we said goodbye and climbed aboard the bike. As we pulled back onto the blacktop highway, the wind rushed back into my face. Tears, not from wind, but from a sad goodbye, flowed down my cheeks, causing my vision to blur. A pressure arose in my chest and throat. I looked back to wave one last goodbye to Muttukadu, to Ramalinga, and to a colorful group of brave children that had received our gifts of caring kindness and given to me a great and enduring treasure.

29

Transformations

Back in Mylapore, Dhamu told me he had a special treat for me. We continued our labyrinthine ride through this street, then that street, eventually arriving at a small temple on the corner of a nondescript street. "Uncle, I know you have a favorite, so I have brought you here to his special place, the temple of Hanuman."

It was a small chapel such as one would find in any city or small town, the indiscriminate site of worship to local devotees or disciples. It had no large courtyards or walls. It was a humble building, almost invisible unless your destination. We rolled into the small lot beside the temple and strolled past a vendor selling flowers, then approached the simple, yet solemn aged stone temple. The aromas of the incense conveyed us within and Dhamu motioned to a priest standing to our left. We approached the priest who, with gladness, entreated us to make our prayers before the deity in the small niche.

Following the flow of other supplicants, we progressed around the temple to other shrines, finishing at the central structure, the key "holy place". Yet a novice, I understood little of figures, but I remembered the instructions of the scholar, that the focus of the supplicant was less-directed at the small statue that was the object of devotion and more to the inner presence of the qualities which that god possessed. I bowed and reflected within as the chants, bells, and smells carried me away.

Though my knowledge of the Hindu pantheon remains scanty, I have, since first learning of him, had an affinity to Hanuman, the great monkey god of Hindu lore. I knew only that he was the devoted aid to Rama in his fight against the great demon Ravana in the Hindu Epic Ramayana and that he had the power to transform himself. While the mighty leader of a great monkey army, he was also able to shrink to the size of a cat to move unnoticed among the enemy camp, or to grow so large he could step from India to Sri Lanka or carry a great mountain in one hand.

I have also had an affinity for monkeys since my childhood. My first attraction was, perhaps, after seeing the movie *Alakazam the Great* when I was about age six. This animated tale followed the odyssey of a small monkey, Alakazam, who desired to become a great and powerful magician. So successful was he that he eventually came to challenge the greatest magician. Due to this act of pride, he was imprisoned in a wasteland. Fortunately, he was saved by the devotion of his sweetheart, whose intrepid love caused her to traverse the wasteland and soften the arrogant heart of the misguided Alakazam. Looking back, somehow that story has presaged my path through life.

An even greater connection to the monkey came during my mime training in the late seventies. I was fortunate to receive training from Tony Montanaro, one of the greats, at the Oklahoma Summer Arts Institute, as earlier reported. Tony put us through regular studio exercises of endless movement scales, physical dialoguing through silent vocabulary with articulation, and illusory action, which allowed us to travel the world in a single spot. Key to Tony's training, however, was not physical prowess, but mental acumen. If we could "become" both internally and externally that which we desired to communicate, we would gain the true mastery of the silent art, to bring the viewer into communion with us in our own transcendent experience.

To gain this ability we were taught to contain the "atmosphere" of our character and gently project it outward. This method was so powerful that decades later, while teaching teens in a gang intervention performance program in Watts, I watched with wonder as students in the balcony identified the character projected by a fellow student on stage with only one or two guesses. There is an emanating cloud that arises from our thoughts and radiates at a great distance from us. While this technique certainly enhances one's presence, I have also found it to be a valuable method to manifest the illusion of invisibility.

The pinnacle of Tony's mental training was the character development technique that he called "I AM", which I referenced regarding my yoga meditation. After a full day of studio technique, we lay supine and exhausted on the studio patio deck facing the lake. Tony began guiding us through a progressive relaxation technique, starting with our toes and following each major muscle group up the body to the top of the head. This is the same method I would later enjoy as the yoga shavasana and a standard hypnotic induction.

Fully relaxing the body and mind and entering a focused waking dream state, we were instructed to imagine a chalkboard upon which was drawn a figure of ourselves. We allowed the self-image to become animated and observed its movement dynamics. We then picked up an eraser and steadily erased the image from the board in our mind. In its place we traced out an image of an animal. In our first exercise, we were given the familiar form of a chimpanzee, whose similar movement structure we had studied.

After drawing the chimp form, we allowed it to become animated and observed every motion from the soles of the feet to the crown of the head. We gave special attention to the way the feet grasped the ground, to the posture of the chest and the movement of the arms in relationship to the movement of the legs. Finally, we focused our attention on the sensory organs of the face: the placement of the ears, the orientation of the nose, the manner of the mouth, and, ultimately, the position and mechanics of the eyes. We looked closely into the eyes, deeper and deeper, until at once, we were looking out through the eyes. We re-oriented ourselves to their perspective, their visual sensibility, and that of the other sensory organs.

After adapting to our new form, we began to explore movement, in time rising up from the floor in characteristic chimp fashion, then engaging in this self-induced animal trance-formation. The urge to explore was irresistible. A curious glint of light reflecting from a scrap of foil on the floor, other crouching forms swaying and swinging, the scent of nature in the breeze, each sensation was experienced in a new way, as danger or food. Lost in my immersion, I only re-oriented as I was bringing a bug to my mouth after a quick olfactory assessment.

The exercise was an awakening for me. I had not known that I could completely lose my sense of self and take on the perceived character with such abandon. It was liberating, and it was a trick I sought to hone to precision. We would take on many animal forms during our studio time, but I eventually found the tool to be useful in projecting myself into the forms of other people in order to mimic their structure, movement, and character.

This method would have profound and lasting impact on me in a spiritual way. After practicing the donning of many individual's ways, like losing my own self-perspective with animals, I also began to observe extra-personal affinity for others. It was as though mentally "walking in others' moccasins" generated a deep sense of empathy and compassion for others. My thinking began to change. I no longer saw myself as separate from others, but only a different track on the same album, each a different expression of the same creative artist.

Further, I was mindful of the night my mentor and youth pastor, Duane Methvin, told the group that we could see the face of God. About sixty of us joined hands in a circle and bowed our heads with eyes closed. Duane told us God had told him that if we followed his instructions we would, indeed, behold the face of God. After a prayer of thanks, we raised our heads and opened our eyes to behold, across the circle, the faces of one another. The exercise left an indelible impression on me and led me to a personal motto to "seek God in every face."

It was, in time, this profound sense of relationship that would turbocharge my desire to help reduce suffering in the world. This connection with the chimp, leading to connection with others, plus my devotion to "know the creator through the contemplation of creation," generated my own mission of compassionate service. That mission had brought me around the world to work with this remarkable community of survivors.

Now, in this meditative prayer, I gave thanks for the transformative power of Hanuman and the invitation to know the ways of others. An extra illumination filled my closed eyes as a surge of uplifting aroma swirled about my head, up my nose, and elevated my mind. I opened my eyes to see the priest before me with the tray of fire and smoke. We smiled at one another as he took some powder from the tray and placed it over my brows.

Dhamu and I clasped hands together and bowed with "Vanakam" and "Nanthree" before turning to exit the temple. Outside, I approached the flower vendor and purchased a strand of small yellow flowers that I draped around my neck. Their fragrance sustained me in the serene state I had been drawn into while praying in the temple as we returned to my room at Ram Guest House.

Once inside my room, with our business arrangements for the following day complete and farewells behind me, I sat in the quiet space, took the flowers from my neck and draped them about the small statue of Ganesha I had purchased in Mamallapuram. I lit a candle and some incense, turned down the lights, picked up my flute, and sat in the sanctuary of my own space, playing a song of gratitude to my beneficent God.

30

Finding the Bell

Daylight was pushing up the dark veil of night as we rode along the beachfront highway en route to another wedding, that of Dhamu's cousin. We passed the lighthouse, which I had seen several times on previous trips. For the first time I was able to observe its light cast out into the bay, guiding vessels, steadfastly standing as a grand guardian of the night. I thought of my Aunt Chee and her affinity for lighthouses. "I must," I thought to myself, "remember to tell her about this one."

We continued south past Srinivasapuram, Adyar, and Besant Nagar, almost to the very edge of the city, already awakened, but coming into view with the increasing light. We arrived at the wedding hall and strolled past a small brass band playing near the entrance. A life-sized Buddha statue stood sentinel at the doorway, blowing bubbles from a fan perched in his up-reaching arms. Inside, the attendees were already seated; we took our place among them.

The ceremony was nearly identical to the previous wedding I had attended and I began to note the significance of the different rites. One of my favorites was the washing and anointing of the feet of the parents by bride and groom. This was a gesture of respect that was not a part of western nuptials, and I appreciated this standard ceremonial element. The band inside, playing drums and pipes, kept the rhythm going throughout the rites. Upon conclusion, we enjoyed a delicious meal of idli, vada, etc., remembering to fold the banana leaf toward us upon completion. We rejoined the family members in the hall as they completed their family gift exchanges, then climbed back aboard the two-wheeler to travel back to town.

We were in the waning days of our time together, wrapping up final visits to those we had provided services to and gathering the gifts that I would take back to the States with me. We returned to the temple in Mylapore to shop in the district around the temple. I was searching for that perfect flute for Sri Latte, plus other items I could take home as souvenirs.

"I must have a bell" I told Dhamudharan. "It should be a small bell that is easy to transport, but must have just the right sound so that when I ring it at times in the future it will have the sweetest sound to remind me of my time in India."

"Uncle, we will find just the right bell for you here, I am certain. They have many things in this area to help people with their prayers."

We stopped first at a small bookstore outside the temple. I was happy to find several books and figurines that would serve as perfect gifts and tokens from this special place. I was even happy to find a copy of Patanjali's *Science of Yoga* at a remarkable price.

As we walked out of the bookstore, I was approached by a sadhu, a holy man clad in meager robes, his face marked with the tilak powder of his prayers. A small spike was protruding about five inches above and below his lower lip, a sign of his spiritual ability to endure suffering. I had read about the sadhus and their spiritual demonstrations that yielded the rewards by which they subsisted. I was a westerner, taking photos of the temple, and clearly a tourist. He stood before me in silent testimony. I offered him some rupees, but remarked to Dhamu that I had seen more impressive piercings on the Venice Beach Boardwalk.

The daylight was reaching that moment of golden hue and its kisses upon the gilded temple caused it to glow in a way I had not seen before. Each of the golden orbs seemed to radiate brilliance in every direction. The carefully sculpted and painted figurines depicting the endeavors of the gods seemed to come to life, as though animated by the brilliance of the sun. I stood watching, captivated by their testimonial, getting a sense that these figurines brought the stories of the Vedas to life for those who attended the temple.

All about the temple, vendors were selling wares; I felt certain there would be a perfect bell on one of the blankets or in one of the stalls lining the adjacent street. Slowly and methodically, I perused each inch, searching for, as a hawk would for a mouse, my treasure. Finally, I found one vendor selling small bells, but the dull tone of each left me continuing my hunt. Facing the street were the numerous shops selling saris, men's clothing, and puja items used in rituals. I prowled through several of the puja shops, but every bell I found, if the proper size, lacked the proper tone. I satisfied myself and a shop owner by purchasing a small silver ceremonial oil lamp.

Nightfall was descending and with it, the need to eat and rest for the next day's project. We stopped at the small restaurant near Ram Guest House that had become our common dining spot. After a small but filling meal, Dhamu delivered me to a browsing center that was still a comfortable walk from the hotel. I called Lenise and had a brief chat about the events of her day and of mine. The time was approaching for my return and our reunion. There were plans to be made. Talking about the details of our soon-to-come time together was both comforting and distressing, knowing that I would soon be with the one I missed so much while in India, while also knowing that I would soon be saying goodbye to this land of mystery and flavor. I completed my call and enjoyed the cool sobering walk back to my room.

While spending time at Srinivasapuram, I had observed the small wooden raft-like kattumarams that the fishermen used to fish nearer to the shore. They were about fifteen feet in length and were constructed from a series of railroad tie sized beams slightly contoured and lashed together. I had spoken with Dhamu about taking a ride on one and he arranged for Vijay to take us out on this Saturday morning.

I rose from bed at my regular hour, as there was no wedding or yoga class to attend. After enjoying my standard light breakfast in my room, I traveled across the street to the browsing center to send some messages while waiting for Dhamu to arrive. To my dismay, I learned that there had been a large aftershock of the initial tsunami-causing earthquake. A tsunami alert had been issued. There was a quiet dread in the air, even in my far-inland location. I immediately contacted as many as I could via email to let them know I was safe. About an hour later, Dhamu arrived and informed me that the village was on alert, but there had been no tsunami; the warning would be lifted in one hour and our journey to sea could proceed with safety.

We arrived in the village to find the tension of the morning easing. People were strolling about and sitting visiting as they would on any casual Saturday. Vijay greeted us and escorted us to the small craft on the beach. The two other fishermen who had joined us on the first boat ride soon arrived and, with our help, began to maneuver the vessel toward the shore. Once in the water, it began to rise, though the small contour caused it to simply rest upon the water, more or less level with the sea, with water rising between the beams to fill the low spaces. We left all but the shorts and shirts we wore on the beach. We helped shepherd the boat to knee-high water and then, following the lead of the others, climbed aboard the swaying planks.

Vijay held one pole at the rear of the boat and another of the men used a pole to push along the bottom, moving the boat further from shore. Once underway, the fellow leaned down and, with one gracefully choreographed move, lifted a wooden block from the deck and with a small lashing, converted his push-pole into a mounted oar. He leaned back against the oar over and over again as Vijay used the other pole to guide the craft. We slipped through the water in a quiet manner, much like paddling out to surf.

After rowing about two-hundred or so yards from shore, the rowing stopped and our quiet drift slowed as the peacefulness of the sea embraced us. The other fisherman, who had been sitting at the front of the catamaran, stood to his feet and leapt from the side of the boat, punctuating the silence with his splash and disappearance beneath the surface. Vijay quickly followed him in, leaping and flipping forward into the sea.

I did not await an invitation. I stood in a similar way, peeling off my shirt as I did, and launched myself, with a similar flipping fashion, off the side of the boat. The sea embraced me and a remarkable sense of surrender, abandon, and liberty rushed over me as I disappeared beneath the surface. I floated freely for just a few moments then rose with a thrust back into the open air. The guys all let out a roaring laugh of celebration, knowing some things, like playing in the water on a Saturday afternoon, transcend language and locale. We were like any lads at any dock near water, enjoying the freedom of play.

Dhamu remained on the skiff. He could not swim. Since he was a child, he told us, his mother would not allow him to go to sea. She had other plans for his life. She began his training in English at an early age so that he might find a different path than the back-breaking labor of the sea. In that mission she had succeeded, but now he could only watch us from the deck of the boat. In our frenzied state of play, this was not acceptable.

Together we gathered around him. "We will help you." We proclaimed. "Come join us in the water." With trepidation he slipped off his shirt and slid slowly from the side of the boat into the water. There was a rope alongside the boat. Vijay gave him the rope to hold and, while taking him by the hand and explaining how to keep himself afloat, began to lead him away from the side of the boat. Then, moving to his other side, he placed himself between Dhamu and the rope, continuing to hold him afloat while giving him a little drift from his anchor. The rest of us swam like a school of fish around him, celebrating his success as we did.

Dhamu's head slipped beneath the water as Vijay continued to hold him in place. Then, as if with a determined proclamation, their hands separated and Dhamu began to stroke and splash in place, independent of any support, save the enthusiasm of his fellows. He treaded in the water for just a few moments then reached out to take the open hand of Vijay. Turning his eyes toward the boat, he released the hand that secured him and splashed exuberantly back to the boat. We let out a collective cheer and swam back to the boat to join him.

We sat together on the soggy boat, soaking the sunshine and resting from our swimming celebration. Each of us recounted our favorite moment, reliving the thrill of the day with each telling. We turned the boat back to shore, but paddled with just a little less vigor than on the ride out.

Once back on the beach, we dragged the craft high on the sand to dry and walked with wobbly sea legs back toward the village. Dhamu told me he had to find a friend on some business and asked that I wait for him. I took a seat on the rubble of Vijay's house and sat drying in the mid-afternoon sun.

Soon a young girl, about 6 or 7 years old approached me. She had been around in previous visits, so we were familiar to each other. She had a plastic character mask, like that worn by children at Halloween, that she had been wearing like a hat on an earlier encounter. Today, she found me alone, quiet, but ready for interruption. She approached with a small paper booklet and presented it to me page-open. On the page was a picture of a bird and beside it a bold word in Tamil. With patient precision, she pointed to the bird and then to the word. "Parima" she said.

"Parima" I replied. And with that my first formal lesson in Tamil began. I had been taught the various phrases and words while together with Dhamu and Vijay, but here was a precious child taking the time with her own materials to help me. Her courage and steady diligence were my greatest lesson as we turned the page to look at more pictures and words.

"Uncle" Dhamodharan's voice rang from the side of the small block house by the beach. I looked up to see him approaching. "I have completed my mission and now we must complete yours." He did not approach me alone, but came walking with his neighbor with whom we had worked regarding his HIV treatment. He was walking with great strength and purpose.

"Thank you" he said. "My life is like before times, happy. Thank you, nanthree." With that he placed his hands together and bowed in the familiar "Vanakam" way. We embrace, two good friends who had been joined in a journey together.

With that, we said goodbye. I stood before our small impromptu beach clinic, a wooden crate covered with an advertising banner as a canopy beside a dark and naked tree. We had been here on this spot. We had done the work. We had seen the healing power that could, transcending word or culture, restore the wounded children of this village. I sighed. Dhamu stood beside me, quietly sharing the same thoughts. Together, we turned and walked back to the two-wheeler. We climbed aboard and, while riding away, I looked back to say my final farewell to Srinivasapuram.

"Uncle, I know one other place that is certain to have what you seek. I will take you there now." Our dinner was complete and the night had arrived, almost my last night in India. We rode from the area near the beach deep within the city. This district was more like a side street of Las Vegas. There were bright lights advertising the many shops along the pedestrian-crowded boulevard. We walked along, part of the crowd, milling, mulling, and finding our way. There were all manner of shops selling the latest fashion wear, electronics, kitchen wares, etc. We entered one shop with a very large open front and an escalator. We stepped aboard the floating staircase and rode to the top.

Once on the second floor, Dhamu directed me to one area of the sprawling warehouse-like shop. There were piles and piles of boxes of different puja items: large standing oil lamps, pots, and trays like those I had seen used in the weddings. I strolled through the aisles until, at last, I came to a shelf of many different sizes and styles of bells. I began to pick them up, one by one, to test their tone. There, in this endless sea of bells, was a small, cleanly cut brass bell. It had a slender stem and atop it was a small animal figure, either a lamb or a calf. I picked it up, admiring its simple elegance. I shook my hand. I heard its light tone, and felt its gentle resonance rest upon my heart. I rang it again and felt my whole soul settle peacefully within. The hurried sound of the shoppers around me drifted out and away in every direction and I stood as though the center of a multi-petaled radiating flower.

I turned to Dhamu. "This is it," I said. "I have found what I was seeking." I rang the bell again and watched for his grin of agreement. With that, I paid the small price at the counter, placed the bell in my pocket, and Dhamu and I made our silent descent back to the street.

31

Hands of God

Dhamu met me at about 5:30 a.m. for another ride, this time on a two-wheeler, through Chennai in the dark. It was my third and final wedding to attend. We rode through the last hour of night, watching the light begin to lift the darkness and reveal the yet-slumbering city. Blackness transitioned to grey and then the golden hues of early morning sun began to shine, opening a brilliant blue canopy above us. The cold wind became less piercing as glints of sunlight began to cast warm channels between the buildings.

In time, we arrived at a large traffic circle. The morning shadows were still casting long shades of grey across the road, but within the shadows were many street people with small straw brooms sweeping the street, creating a clean motorway. In Los Angeles, this ritual would be performed by the fleet of street-sweeping machines with their familiar whirring brushes. Along with the cleaned gutters came the weekly threat of a large parking fine. Here, however, a similar outcome was produced by the diligence of persons who had, in their nightly huddles on sidewalks, seemed like castaways in the urban sea. Today, on this fresh morning, I saw that it was they who prepared the city for each day, and whose common pleas for rupees for tea were an earned reward to be offered with gratitude.

We drove on as if the city would never end, riding for over one hour through neighborhood after neighborhood until at last the city began to thin in a similar manner as to the south near Muttukadu. Dhamu, still stopping to check the address on the invitation with different buildings, continued toward the site of his friend's wedding. Eventually, as the city nearly disappeared altogether, we arrived at a small building beside the road.

The wedding was not scheduled to begin for another half hour. Across the road from the pavilion was a small lake. We climbed from the two-wheeler and walked to the lake as the cool morning began to warm with the rising sun.

Now that I was off the bike and walking toward the lake, I recognized a different quality to the air. It was that sense of freshness one experiences when traveling from the city to the country. My lungs seemed to reach for more air and be more refreshed by what I received. We strolled along a small paved walkway across the dam that formed the lake.

While taking in the country morning, we were met by Vijay and another of Dhamu's friends who had also come for the wedding. We gleefully greeted one another then journeyed back across the road to attend the ceremony. When we reached the pavilion we were met by Dhamu's mother and sisters, who had arrived via autorickshaw. We all entered the building together and took our seats as Dhamu's mother and sisters went to the platform to participate in the ceremony.

During this ceremony I began to observe the now-familiar rituals: the groom's pouring of ghee over the small fire in the bowl before the couple and the priest, the gold pieces tied with string across the foreheads of the bride and groom, the cleansing of the parents' feet, the passing of the coconut around the room for blessings and gatherings of rice, the pitching of rice upon the bride and groom on cue, and the placement of the ring on the second toe of the bride by the groom.

After the ceremony, I followed the parade down the stairs to the dining hall. Just before the entrance to the hall was the door to the kitchen. I looked in to behold the behind-the-scenes preparation of the feast. Giant stew pots were being stirred on large fires, while one gentleman ladled batter onto a large griddle to produce dosas, the crepe-like wraps that were used to gather veggies or sop sauce. I took my place with Dhamu at the long table and enjoyed the parade of "bucketeers" who poured round after round of deliciousness onto my banana leaf. With both satisfaction and sorrow I folded my leaf toward me to say "enough," though I still wanted more of the splendid feast.

After presenting gifts to the bride and groom, Dhamu and I joined several of his schoolmates in the yard in front of the pavilion. As I stood near the road, I was enchanted by the scene of several cows that had come to the pavilion and were feasting on the remnants of the meals, along with the banana leaves, that had been left by attendees and deposited into a large trough by the kitchen workers. The colorful ribbons festooning the trough area made it seem as though the cows were the final celebrants of the wedding festival.

As I stood admiring the feasting cows, my attention was redirected by an approaching throng of ducks. From behind the small building next to the trough emerged a cavalcade of ducks, about two-hundred or more, walking directly toward me. As I did not have time to move, the approaching wave of ducks parted around me and progressed nonplused by my presence. Behind the ducks was their driver, a Tamil fellow wearing a short lungi and carrying a stick with a colorful rag dangling from the end that he used to herd the ducks in a mass as they proceeded onward. It was a grand and surreal conclusion to a strange and blessed morning.

We climbed back aboard the two-wheeler to embark on our next adventure. Vijay joined us with Dhamu's nephew Jodash sitting astride the motorcycle gas tank, hands grasping the handlebar crossbar. We rolled through the Chennai traffic, now heavier in the late Sunday morning. Dhamu told me he had a special treat for me. At one intersection we parted ways with Vijay as he headed back to Srini.

We rode on to a bridge-like outlook from which we could see a massive rail yard and gargantuan shipping container cranes. It was the Port of Chennai and Dhamu took pride in showing me this great wonder, one of the largest in the world. I could not see the full port, however, only a monolithic wall of stacked containers that blocked my view of the water. It was not an unfamiliar view, as I had seen the Port of Los Angeles many times and from this perspective, despite the aged railcars, the view was much the same.

Continuing our trek, we arrived at a nearby apartment building and Dhamu climbed from the bike and called to an upper window. A voice called back down with a degree of surprised enthusiasm. We were met at the door with a warm greeting and taken back up to the apartment of an older couple, delighted to see Dhamu and meet his foreign friend.

As we sat in the comfortable living room, a tale unfolded. The woman was Dhamu's English teacher when he was young. His mother had sought her help to teach Dhamu English in order to give him greater options in life than the family tradition of fishing. With dreamy reminiscence, she told us how Dhamu was, since that early age, devoted to learning and becoming the person his mother had wanted him to be.

Other family members joined us and we discussed the project, my life in Los Angeles, and the therapeutic and musical interests we shared. At some time during the conversation, I realized that we were all speaking English, that it was not necessary to translate the conversation back and forth. This, though a seemingly simple thing, was like a sweet retreat within a sea of foreign language, giving me a sense of restfulness. We enjoyed some drinks together, sharing tales of all our lives flowing from different channels to arrive at this pool of hospitality.

Further along our journey, we stopped at the home of another friend, Adul Khader. We met him at the door, where we were asked to remove our shoes. We entered the small apartment that had no furniture and were invited to sit on the floor. This, Dhamu told me, was a Muslim home, whose traditions were different than the others we had been in. We sat together for about half an hour, getting to know one another and discussing our project, as we had on the visits with others. During the conversation, Dhamu explained how their friendship had remained strong for many years despite their different religious traditions.

It was mid-afternoon when we finally returned to the Guest House. We made plans to meet early in the evening to try again to find a flute for Sri Latte. I took advantage of the break to begin my packing. It was my last full day and night in India. Tomorrow's schedule promised to be very full, so I began to organize my bags and get things ready to go so I could enjoy the day to its fullest.

We met again just after dark and began our trek to find a flute at the Tamil Nadu State Fair. We rode through the Chennai night with schoolboy excitement. Dhamu was excited not just at the prospect of discovering our long-sought treasure, but at showing me the splendor of India at the fair.

While sitting at one light, he pointed to riders on a bike beside us. "Uncle, notice how these two have covered their faces." Indeed, the two riders wore scarves across their faces so that only their eyes were visible. "They have made a promise to be secret loves," Dhamu reported. "They will only allow their faces to be seen by each other and no-one else."

I looked back at the riders, here in the sea of people packed along their way. They were one set of riders on one two-wheeler in a sea of two-wheelers, auto-rickshaws, cars, trucks, etc. Yet, somehow, they were still in their own cloistered lovers' embrace. I took some pleasure in their secret pact, knowing that they were demonstrating the power of romantic love for all of us. Though thousands of miles away, I instantly felt the clutch of my not-so-secret lover in the hidden chambers of my heart.

There was a great glowing brown fog around the entrance to the Fair. Car lights blazed through the dust stirred by constant coming and going, while the channa masala carts sent their smoke rising to carry the enticing aromas to would-be patrons. We found an appropriate parking spot and joined the flowing crowd into the gates. My eyes scoured the environment as we went from booth to booth looking at all manner of enticing treat, the ornamentations of life: bangles, saris, hair clips, even henna tattoo sets danced before me in their bins. There were games to play, foods to enjoy, entertainment in tents and on the street, and even rides as at any county or state fair. Familiar also, was the throng of people within which we all moved as a mass. My greatest enjoyment was at a horticultural tent. I saw the most elegant orchids and other unique flowers; I photographed them to share with Lenise.

Alas, however, there was no flute for me. Having searched the entire fair, we decided to leave. It was getting late and the fair would soon close, so we made our way back to the two-wheeler. As we approached the exit, we saw a vendor standing by the gate holding a pole on which, like fruit on a tree, were hanging many different toys. There, amidst the toys, on the staff held by the vendor we likely passed on the way in, was the ideal bamboo beginner's flute. I took one flute from the stand and began to play. It was perfect. It played without effort and invited me to find its song. With glee and a profound sense of completion, I purchased two of the flutes, one for Sri Latte and one for my grandson Tobin.

We were quite exhausted by the time I was returned to the Hotel. I made arrangement with Dhamu to meet early in the morning then went to my room to rest for the night. I had enjoyed seeing the full moon rising during the ride home, so after I settled back into the room, I decided to go to the rooftop and enjoy this on my last night in Chennai. I took my flute and climbed to the rooftop patio. The city was still filled with its never-ending noise, but in the still moment of night, I sat and played my song of fulfillment. I played with thankfulness for the success of the trip. I played for the opportunity that had now been realized. I played for the beauty of the villagers who had shown such dignity in the midst of turmoil. I played for the long-desired dream that was now becoming a memory.

After playing for some time, I opened my eyes and realized I was not alone. In the moonlight, I could see a figure sitting some distance from me that had not been there when I came out to play. It was the room attendant who had brought me my hot bathing water during the previous nights. He had also stopped by my room on a couple of occasions to discover what new flute I had acquired and even made attempts to play a couple of them.

"I do not want to disturb you or stop your playing" he said. "I only heard you and thought it would be nice to sit and listen."

"Come then, let's sit together," I said, and invited him to sit nearer to me. We sat together in the peacefulness of the night. "I am just trying to gather these last moments of my last night in Chennai. Tomorrow I return to America"

"Oh," he said, "then I have a gift I would like to give to you, but I will need to travel to my home in the morning to get it. It is a small statue of a flute-player that I have painted myself. I would like to make it a gift to you, because you are the real flute-player who has been my friend."

"Thank you," I said. "I look forward to receiving such a thoughtful gift."

"Do you feel that your time here has been successful for you?" he asked.

"Oh yes," I said "beyond anything I could have imagined. I did not know what to expect when we came, only that I wanted to help the people who were tsunami-affected."

"I think that you have made a great success here," he said. "I am happy that you have come and I have made a friend from America, but the people are most happy that you have come. Do you know what it is meaning to them that you have come here? It means everything to them.

"When tsunami came, we were all like lost children. We were crying out to God saying 'please save us; please help us from this terrible tsunami.' But God does not have feet that he can walk among us, and

God does not have hands that he can reach out and touch us. But you have feet, and with those feet you have come here to walk among us, and you have hands and with your hands you have reached out and touched us. This is why the people are so thankful to you. They feel that you are the answer to their prayers, that God sent you to help us and you have."

A sort of numbness struck me, and beyond that a sense of fullness that rose to become a satisfied smile. "Thank you," I said. "That means everything to me. I have come from the desire of my heart to help those who suffer, bringing the abilities I have learned to help make a difference. It is my true delight to know that we have been part of something so special."

Suddenly, many of the images of our treatments flashed through my mind, the comments of the villagers when we asked to place hands on them, and particularly the veiled acceptance of the injured woman outside the temple when I gave treatment. I was only a stranger to them, but the grace that flowed through me was very familiar.

The bright moon still smiled down upon us as though the moment would not end. I brought the flute to my lips and played another song of thanks.

32

The List

I woke early to enjoy my last day in India. The light was increasing, though the sun was not quite up as I rose, dressed, and crossed the street to attend my final yoga session with Sri Latte.

By now I had become a familiar member of the group and knew the routine. I climbed the quiet staircase to the rooftop, acquired a small rug from the collection by the door, walked over to a place in the center of the rooftop, unrolled the rug, sat, and began to meditatively limber up my body and mind. Sri Latte took her place before us and began to guide us through some simple pranayama.

We continued through what was now a familiar cycle of movement, my mind focused not on my ability to realize this posture or that, but in the simple enjoyment of the effort. I knew that I was breathing the air, hearing the stirring of the city, and following the guidance of my instructor in concert with the simple inflow and outflow of my breath. Our asanas complete, I welcomed the quiet rest of shavasana and waited for the permissive command to "set my mind free like a kite on a long string." In my stillness, I floated high above the hospital, the street, the city, and India. I hovered there, taking it all in, holding it close, as though breathing it in to every cell. When the meditation was complete, I lingered, savoring the moments with my whole being, as one would the delicious and enduring flavors of a treasured meal.

When I finally stirred and began to return my rug to the pile, I was given warm farewells from my fellow attendees who exited the rooftop with a hurried calm. I waited for Sri Latte to complete her business before inviting her to the shaded area of the roof where we had conducted our previous flute lesson. She sat with schoolgirl excitement for her second lesson. Once settled, I produced the flute that I had purchased at the fair and, holding it toward her, said "my gift to you."

Her eyes leapt with delight as she reached out to take the flute, receiving it like a treasure and examining it as she held it in her hands. She brought it to her lips, carefully placing her fingers over the holes, and blowing out a low and soothing tone. She lifted each finger tentatively to hear the next note, repeating a few to make sure she got it right. When she was finished, she took the flute from her lips, moved her hand along its smooth surface, drew it toward her as in an embrace and said "thank you, this will work perfectly for me, you must have searched far to find such a lovely flute."

I related the story of my search and my gladness to find it on a path I had already traveled. I then produced the second flute I had purchased for Tobin and said "now let us play some music together."

I lifted the flute to my lips and encouraged her to do the same. I waited until she had settled the fingers securely in place then slowly began to lead her in playing the scale. She followed along as we both beamed our happiness through our stereophonic tone. We played up, then down the scale, her finger placement becoming more confident as she listened to the notes we were producing. I encouraged her to practice every day, and then showed her how to play a very simple tune by simply changing the timing by which she played each note. She mimicked my playing perfectly.

After about thirty minutes, our time together had come to an end. She invited me in to her treatment office and offered me a gift of a poster of yoga postures specifically recommended for back care, according to the medical application of yoga common in India. We thanked one another again for the exchange of gifts, not just the flute and poster, but the shared instruction that left us both feeling as though we had given something and received something, the perfect foundation of friendship. We embraced, faced one another, and holding hands together bowed our salute "Vanakam."

I left her office and descended the staircase with somber serenity, taking each step with peaceful pleasure. I walked out of the hospital and onto the busy street. A full day awaited me.

The previous night I had compiled a list of the errands necessary to complete my final day in India. At the top of the list was sending a report back to the States. I slipped into the browsing center, took my seat at my now-familiar station, and composed my third and final Field Report. I transferred my remaining photos from my digital camera and produced a disc of the over eight-hundred photographs. The staff of the small center had become like close friends. We, too, said our goodbyes, and I crossed the street to return to my room and complete my packing.

Soon, Dhamu arrived bringing a small package to add to my bags. The pants that I had purchased during my first days had a faulty seam that had separated. I had sent them to be repaired by the tailor for whom we had purchased the sewing machine. I was happy to be both a patron of the machine and a patron of the craft. Dhamu had also taken some of my clothing for laundering in the village and they, along with the newly restored pants, were bundled like a gift. I opened the package and carefully arranged the fresh items in my bag.

Leaving the bags in my room staged for departure, we boarded the two-wheeler and set out on our day's endeavors. Our first stop was at the local Western Union office. Our requests for funding assistance, along with updated reports, had yielded dynamic results with many friends sending money to support the work. The funds received would be the final payment for Dhamodharan. Our accounts settled, we set out toward our next stop.

I had been particularly delighted by a specific song I heard on the radio during our travels, "Khadal Vhala Thein" which was a song from the Tamil Super 8 film "Manmadhan". We arrived at the music store and immediately located the soundtrack CD. Dhamu also recommended several other CD's of Tamil Village Music and Indian music luminary A.R. Rahman. We were still close to the Ram Guest House, so we dropped the music by before heading to the favored temple plaza in Mylapore.

The glasses I had ordered were waiting when I returned to the shop. They needed very little adjustment and Dhamu was patient in his waiting. Afterward, we crossed the street to return to the familiar restaurant, this time to relish one more Special Thali Meal. We took a seat at the back of the air-conditioned room and gave the waiter our order. Instantly, a banana leaf was placed on the table and the pageant of culinary extravagance began: a pile of rice, ghee, relishes, sauces, etc., over and over again. We reviewed our project and revisited each successful moment between every delicious mouthful. Our work was done. Dhamu would need to follow up with the villagers we had worked with, but we celebrated the splendid outcomes we had achieved.

"Uncle" Dhamodharan said. "There is another Tamil word I would like you to know. It is 'anna'. It is a name one uses to speak to his older brother. I would like to now call you 'Anna'."

"That is wonderful, and what is the name for a younger brother?" I asked.

"That is 'tambi'." He answered. "You would say 'yin tambi', meaning 'my little brother'."

"Ok then," I said, "from now on you will be yin Tambi!"

"Ok, Anna." Dhamu replied.

Besides the farewell dinner later with Dhamu's family, there was still one thing for me to experience before leaving India. Two months earlier, while in Los Angeles prepping for our trip to Guatemala, I had a strange dream. In the dream, Lenise and I were in a train station. I was surprised because the station was not in Guatemala, but in India. The station was crowded with travelers as I had seen perhaps in a Roland Joffe film or documentary. People were piling things on top of the train and climbing aboard for departure. We were waiting for Mitta to arrive, because she was going to accompany me on the train.

The images and smells were remarkably vivid. The sense of urgent expectancy was visceral. This dream occurred before the earthquake and tsunami, before we knew I would go to India, and with Mitta. When I awoke, I told Lenise the dream. We both knew that it was some portend. I knew that before leaving India it was important that I take a ride on a train.

The train depot was just a block from the temple square. Basker and Vijay met us there. In the late afternoon, pre-rush hour, the depot was sparsely populated, open and airy. We purchased tickets for a brief ride and boarded a nearly empty train car. It was a commuter train, not the long distance train I had seen in film or in my dream, but when it began to roll out from the station, my imagination moved with it.

We rode out above the city on elevated tracks, looking down upon the activities on the street such as those we had recently been a part of. On one street a wedding was taking place and young men were dancing about on the street. We leaned out of the open doors of the train and saw others in adjacent cars doing the same.

As we crossed over the river, I looked down to see one approaching bank of the river speckled with multi-colored grave sites with crosses. I knew this to be a Christian cemetery, but Dhamu told me, to my surprise, that there were Hindu graves also. Cremation was a special ceremony only for persons who had completed certain temple rites during life.

As we cruised over the river, I noticed a veritable village of small thatched huts filling the flood plain right up to the water's edge. They would be carried away by any serious flood of this river. The poor here, living in the most meager dwellings in the most marginal of environments, remained at the highest risk for suffering. I expressed my concern for them to Dhamu as we passed.

We encountered several stops along the way, the train car filling at each stop until, at last, it filled to brimming. When we arrived at the end of the line, the train emptied again, then repeated the same cycle on its return. We disembarked at the familiar station with one of the final checkmarks made to the list.

We returned to the hotel to load my bags into the auto and set out for my final dinner at Dhamu's house. Along the way, Dhamu reported that there was one important errand he wanted to make. He informed Basker and Vijay of his desire to purchase a poster of Sai Baba to send to Jim Uncle. We arrived at the temple and Dhamu quickly identified a stall that was selling the poster.

He purchased the poster and was returning it to the auto when I noticed a crowd of devotees standing before the temple. One of them approached me, asking for rupees for tea. I reached into my pocket and gave him a two-rupee coin. Others, seeing my giving, began to approach. I produced two twenty rupee notes from my pocket and asked Vijay to go to a vendor and change it to two-rupee coins. He returned with a handful of coins and I approached the crowd, giving a coin to as many as I could, saluting each with "Vanakam" as I did. I would like to have purchased tea for all in the crowd, for all of India. Instead, I provided all I could at the time, before being carted away for one final family feast.

We arrived at Dhamu's family's home with all of the fanfare that had accompanied every other visit. I was greeted upon entry by each of the family members. Dhamu's mother promptly took me to the back room to make prayers at the family altar; she then applied the red powder to my forehead.

We returned to the front room; Dhamu's sisters were already setting up the mat on the floor where we would sit for my meal. Tonight, Subathra had made a special effort to prepare chapattis and channa masala. I ate with delight and gratitude, each bite eliciting sighs of pleasure. Every time the volume of food on the plate was diminished, she would ladle another portion of the dark, creamy, chickpea treat. I ate, and ate, and ate, thinking I could not contain another bite, but knowing each bite intensified the pleasure for all of us. When I was finished, I picked up the small banana on a separate plate and began to enjoy the cooling treat of completion.

I sat back against the wall, fully sated. The trays were cleared and another sense of excitement arose. Deepash stepped forward and sat before me with a small package, lifted it toward me with both hands and looking directly into my eyes, said "my gift to you." I met his reach and received the small plastic box, opened it, and marveled at the various trinkets and bobbles contained within.

"For your wife, Uncle," Dhamodharan said. Each of the sisters also presented me with a gift, saying "my gift to you."

I thanked them for the gifts and all of the hospitality they had provided, then said "I will leave you with the one unique gift I have, a song from my flute." I pressed the flute to my lips and began to play a song of sad farewell, filled with rolling adventure and discovery. While playing, we all were as one. I recalled Dhamu's curiosity at the flute when I first produced it, wondering how this flute could make a difference for his people, seeing how this flute was now making its difference in the room, creating a moment, a mood, a manner that would imprint our time together, giving tone to the song we had crafted during my visit. My playing complete, I rested the flute on my lap, raised hands together and said to each, "Nanthree, Vanakam."

There was one last bit of business for Dhamu and I to complete. We sequestered ourselves in the back room with my portable recorder so I could conduct a project completion interview. In the dimly lit room he recounted his tsunami experience, his voice breaking at several points throughout the account.

"Before tsunami, the situation for many in my village was critical. Six of ten in the village made their living from the sea, others from working in the market selling the fish. For them, there was no sense of time, only the conditions of the sea. When the signs were right, they would go out on the sea to catch fish. This was their life, their only way to provide for their families. On the 26th, the day of tsunami, all that was lost, all boats and nets broken and dragged out to the deep sea.

"Each family was in its home, as it was a holiday. When the wave came there were only seconds to act. One second the waves came in to the house and my family fled to the floor above, the next second the wave went out and carried away all of the things that we had. Not only icebox, photos, and clothes, but also the jewels saved for my sisters' weddings were gone, carried away by the sea.

"Many of the children, aged 12 to 16, were playing cricket on the field when the wave came. My friend told me he could hear their cries as they fought the wave, but could not help. We lost many children, some very young, 11 months, 4 months old only. One woman, married only one month, lost her husband to the tsunami. The bodies of the dead were scattered all around and people were walking with no clothes, only dressed like a just-born baby. All of the brightness of their life was gone.

"It took me twelve hours to find my family. Our situation was now very critical. We had nothing and no way to get the things that we needed. It was only because of the kindness of my friends who brought blankets, food, and eventually gave a place to stay and wash that my whole family was saved. Soon after, thanks to Jim Uncle and others who were like gods to us, we began to receive help. Money was sent to help the children to have books and uniforms for their education. This is the most critical thing for the people, that the children can get an education to provide the things that are needed for their families without having to go to the sea.

"Then Jim Uncle said that he is sending two friends to help who will need my guidance. I began to think of how I might help the people of my village, how I might use the help of these foreigners to help the people of my whole area. I made a plan then to help many of the people who are tsunami-affected.

"When you came, at first I did not understand how you would help with a flute. I know my people, that they are looking for something, and I am wondering why you came to India to only play a flute. Then I began to think, 'no, there is something to learn from you that will be useful to our people.'

"After learning of your treatments, I have become very impressed with this work. I have learned many things about my people. If you give them money, you will be giving and giving and giving, and this can become a problem for them, creating many misunderstandings. But giving the treatment, we are helping them to do something for themselves. This First Medicines is something very precious. It is like feeding energy to a child, showing the calmness place to entire India.

"I am very thankful. Not only from me, I hear many thanks from those whom we have given treatment. They are now very glad through First Medicines. I give many thanks to Jim Uncle for giving this great opportunity to learn the human calmness. I am thankful to you for Jim Uncle sending you here to help us to learn these treatments.

"What is the advantage of this First Medicines to our people is a high percentage of our people are uneducated. I particularly like your treatment because it is simple to learn not only for educated, but you have created a treatment for poor people, for the uneducated people. Thank you for doing this and bringing it to us. This is not an ending, this is a beginning.

"We worked a lot of cases, especially I remember working with my friend who was affected by AIDS. Through your treatment he is now feeling very happy, very happy with his family, and all the people can see this success. We have lightened one family's brightness and through that many others will be happy. Then, we went to Muttukadu. We gave a lot of treatment for the child and she has improved much. We went to Cuddalore and taught a lot of people this training. Especially, we have given good sleep for every tsunami-affected person who received treatment from us. This was our success.

"Whatever lesson I have observed through working with First Medicines I will implement. I will use this formula. Not only is it a formula, it is a medicine; not only a medicine, it is a love, a love medicine that I will implement. We have created self-confidence for the body, how to help the body heal, how to remove the sadness. It was not a lie, it is the truth, I have spoken to many of the people we have treated.

"If I see any person declaring his problem, I will give this First Medicines treatment. To this person I will say 'these are simple methods, they are "user-friendly", be calm, calm, calm; find your safe place. While you are breathing out your sadness and all those things are coming out, while you are taking the breath inside, the powerful medicines, the energy is flowing to all the parts of the body, each part is going to receive all of the goodness. While we are touching your arms and legs, we are removing your sadness, be happy, be happy."

Night had arrived while we were dining, and with it darkness. Vijay already had my bags loaded into the waiting autorickshaw. Basker sat ready to drive. I said my goodbyes to the family; Dhamu and I climbed aboard. In the dark alleyway, I could not really make out the company standing in the shadows, but I held my flashing camera in their direction and captured an image of the sentinels of farewell, standing with somber faces, saying goodbye to their friend from America.

We traveled through the familiar roadways. They too were friends I would embrace while passing. Dhamodharan and I continued our discussion of the project continuation as we traveled. The long, lighted city drive finally ended at the airport departure lanes. We loaded my bags onto a cart. I said my farewells to the guys and took my place in line to enter the airport terminal. I checked my bags then changed some rupees for dollars. I felt as though I had passed through a web, stepped out of a time machine, and exited my cloistered mission. I stepped into a restroom to refresh myself and as I washed my face, I watched the red color disappear into the drain.

The airport announcer's chant-like voice set a cadence to my steps as I steadily plodded my way to the gate. The waiting area was nearly full, but I found a small row of seats alone, facing the window onto the walkway to the plane. I took my seat and nestled my backpack between my legs. As I sat, I looked through the glass. On the other side of the glass was my world. In moments I would traverse that lane to begin my journey home. In this bustling realm, with what time remained, I closed my eyes to hold on to the dream.

Epilogue

A young male cardinal is perched on the birdbath outside my home-office window. His feathers have not yet turned red, but his crown feathers rise to reveal his distinctive profile as he darts to chase the blue-jays and sparrows away. Flowering cannas stand tall in the borders of the freshly-planted garden beds as Tibetan prayer flags sway in the gentle breeze on this mild, overcast June day in Oklahoma. Almost ten years have passed since I first sat to record the story of my Indian Tsunami odyssey, years of review and remembrance, of coming to understand the mystery of the healing miracles I observed.

When I returned to Los Angeles, Mitta brought me an article she had discovered in a magazine after her return. It was written by a physician with Doctors Without Borders working in Thailand during the same time we were in India. He reported that they had brought bandages and medicines to help the tsunami victims, but found injuries they were not prepared to treat. He told of their sleeplessness, loss of appetite, diverse pains, and tremors at the word "tsunami", the exact conditions we had seen successfully resolved.

I pondered why our treatments had been so successful. I had every confidence in the hypnotic recovery methods employed, but was surprised by the speed and stability by which those we had treated regained their sense of balance. I reviewed the dynamics of the interventions. Perhaps it was the overwhelming stimulus that we provided by treating head, heart, hands, and feet while guiding through emotional restoration. This became an equal and opposite supportive response to the destructive force of the tsunami. An undeniable element in our interventions was the reported perception that they were "touched by a god", itself a potent comprehensive medicine.

Our methods were clinical and rooted in my own practice ethic to keep matters of faith and spirituality out of the therapeutic environment unless introduced by the client. I was trained to "deal with what emerges," so when religious traditions are brought forward, I try to support them in the best way I can. India is a land steeped in spiritual tradition. Religious devotion infuses every aspect of life. It was inescapable that complete healing would require support of body, mind, *and* spirit.

This is the dividend that the work in India brought to First Medicines. Our physical and psychological interventions were effective; however, there was an extra element, the sense that they were being helped by something beyond themselves, more powerful, fueling whatever capability they found within. This is not a discovery, only an observation. This faith, or "G-factor", in healing is as old as humanity; it is the first medicine.

Soon after my return, I developed a plan to promote the same benefits far and wide. I wrote a script that included all of the release and restoration suggestions that had been effective in India. I titled the brief script "The Five Minute Miracle" and printed it on 5x7 postcards with which I could "paper the world" to make it as ubiquitous as the American Sign Language cards I have appreciated since my childhood.

Some months later, after teaching a workshop on Emergency Hypnosis, I found myself at the airport in Dallas, Texas making a hurried return to Los Angeles ahead of a hurricane approaching the Gulf Coast. Hours later I watched in horror as New Orleans became swamped by Hurricane Katrina. Ten months passed before I had the opportunity to go to New Orleans to offer help. After teaching the same emergency course near Denver, I was invited by attendee and nurse-hypnotherapist Brenda Fister to join the Emergency Communities relief encampment in St. Bernard Parish, a district of New Orleans that was seriously impacted. By this time, what began as a devastating flood had become an enduring torment.

For ten days I made my five-mile drive through the still-decimated landscape of the Lower Ninth Ward and St Bernard Parish to arrive at the great domed refuge. Emergency Communities was established by a group of young people, including Brenda's daughter and son-in-law, who felt compelled to offer help to the people of the area. Soon after the hurricane, they began offering three warm meals a day, an internet café, medical care, clothing, household and cleaning supplies, plus a comfortable place to simply find some peace. The camp was also populated by many young people who had traveled to the area to help those in need "muck out" their houses and put their lives back together again.

Upon arrival I began to scope-out the environment to determine how we might be able to offer help. In a large teepee, volunteers gathered to learn how they could discharge their stress and help others with "The Five Minute Miracle". To my satisfaction, the next day two young women reported that the bugs and noise of the refrigerator truck engines had kept them awake every night. After employing the instructions to "allow every sound to carry you deeper into relaxation," the same sounds had serenaded them into their best sleep since first pitching their tents.

Reaching out to the locals who were coming through the camp was a different story. Where we had a couple of hours to conduct a clinic in each of the villages in India, here that appeared to be a vast volume of time, which would only add stress by limiting their activity time. We needed a different intervention that would be appropriate to this setting. My years of experience as a nightclub and street performer came to my aide. During an afternoon of observation of the flow of traffic, I located a spot where attendees had extra time, the chow line.

Before leaving Oklahoma City, where Lenise and I had relocated to be closer to family, I had recorded a CD of "The Five-Minute Miracle" to help out a friend. I had a copy of that CD with me, along with a folding recliner I brought in order to conduct full hypnosis sessions. I found a spot about halfway down the 200ft line that would allow people to feel they had plenty of time before arriving at the serving area. There, I set up a relief station, complete with a cardboard and marker sign that read "Stressed? Take Five".

My first recipient sat in the chair with a cloud of uncertainty that affected us all. I reclined her in the chair, placed headphones on her, and turned on the player. While listening, I began giving a hands-on treatment using standard Reiki hand positions from head to toe, with a few extra areas treated according to my new understanding of acupuncture points. I gently embraced my passive charge, giving intention to each flowing touch, and completed the treatment by playing flute as the recording concluded. To our amazement, when the recording ended and the "client" opened her eyes, a broad smile helped broadcast the remarkable relief she had received. I had discovered an intervention method that allowed a person in a folding recliner, next to a meal line, in a parking lot, in a disaster zone to experience bliss in just over six minutes.

We repeated the treatment over and over, three meals a day for the next ten days. Astonishingly, the responses were almost universal. The most remarkable outcome was an elderly gentleman who, during our post-treatment chat, remarked "yesterday I told my wife I couldn't take it anymore, that I was ready to put a gun in my mouth and end it. Now I feel like I can move on." I saw one young fellow limping across the camp and invited him for a treatment. He said he had hurt his foot while playing basketball and had just come from the Medical Tent but was still in a great deal of pain. Seven minutes later, his pain was gone. We were both impressed.

Since that time, I have made it the central outreach of First Medicines to provide "Five-Minute Miracle Free Stress Relief Treatments" at public events. I have provided hundreds of interventions at Health Food Stores, Health and Business Expos, and Street Fairs. Mostly, individuals open their eyes and remark how wonderfully relaxing the experience was for them. Occasionally after treatment, I will receive a report of the remarkable distress or pain they were experiencing and their profound sense of relief, comfort, and optimism upon completion. I have called this my seining net, for in offering broad relief to any, I have had the chance to provide meaningful relief to some whose needs were critical.

After news of other disasters to which we could not travel, I posted video instruction on our website, firstmedicines.org, along with the recording and written script for individuals to access through this internet portal. Following the violence of the Arab Spring, we posted a version in Arabic and in response to events in the Philippines and Japan, have also posted versions in Spanish and Japanese.

We also utilized the internet to deliver a series of trainings via Skype for workers in the field hospitals near Tahrir Square in Cairo. I adapted the Emergency Hypnosis protocols for First Responders as "Critical Care Communication". Pierre-Etienne Vannier worked as First Medicines Arab States Coordinator and set up the trainings with both Christian and Muslim groups and facilitated the class in Cairo; I taught from my office in Oklahoma City. Etienne subsequently relocated to Los Angeles and has resumed the HIV/AIDS Initiative there.

In May of 2013, a massive tornado passed eight miles from my home. It destroyed much of Moore, Oklahoma. In the days following, I worked directly with the medical relief team at the Moore First Baptist Church. The Five Minute Miracle Stress Relief station became an integral part of the care given to both survivors and relief workers. The doctors also brought me into the exam and treatment areas to play flute for the distressed victims.

I spent one day with the medical team going door-to-door in Little Axe, a rural community that was also decimated by a tornado the day before the Moore event. Doctor Laura Asher was very keen on having me play my flute during meetings with residents who needed care. I also found creative ways to deliver The Five Minute Miracle.

I observed the importance of spiritual medicine in this community. We visited a woman who was in hospice care at her trailer home. After being checked out medically and given the tools of The Five Minute Miracle and a strand of beads for The Coué method to help with her neuropathic pain, she spoke of her faith and invited prayer according to Christian tradition. Nearby, an old Indian man endured his check-up to the sounds of my flute then told us of his traditional ways and how he had spoken to the angry wind when it passed. He also recited a Cherokee prayer for us.

I have maintained regular contact with Dhamodharan. In the days and weeks following our visit, he made many presentations at schools and other groups about the work we had done and the importance of implementing these "first medicines". The challenging life that existed before the tsunami has continued. He has maintained the support of his family, providing the marriage arrangements for both of his sisters who were unmarried at the time of our visit. He has even welcomed a new niece to the family. He also faced the demand of financing hospital care for his father when his health began to decline, and eventually the provision of funeral arrangements after his death. He has been working in sales and management and has recently obtained a law degree.

Dhamu's greatest challenge came after seriously injuring his shoulder in a motorcycle accident. He experienced severe nerve damage that limited his ability to use his right hand. He used his "strongbody" methods, along with physical therapies, and has almost regained full function. He reports that all those we worked with in his village continue to report good outcomes, including his friend with AIDS who claims his life is still happy "like before times."

Mitta returned to India some months after our trip to help the family of the single woman and daughter repair the roof of their house. She has become involved in other service organizations in India. Basker took a job in the Arab States soon after our time together in India, but has now returned to Tamil Nadu. Vijay and his "would-be" were married in the year after our visit and have since become parents. Mitta, Jim, and I raised funds to help provide a new boat, motor, and nets for him.

After returning from India, Lenise and I moved from Los Angeles to Oklahoma City, living in the same neighborhood as when we met in 1983. This has allowed us more frequent visits with my parents and our grandsons Tobin and Jasper. I worked for five years as director of Oklahoma Healing Arts Institute and studied, acupuncture, Chinese dietary therapy, reflexology, aromacology, and homeopathy. I have incorporated these into my practice and services menu of First

Medicines, including as elements of the Five Minute Miracle Treatment. I now maintain private practice in a quiet office suite in an atrium garden building that is a ten minute walk from our home. I continue to travel to teach and conduct outreach.

My flute, its own character in the India story, has since gone on to travel the world as part of Mayan Shaman Tata Pedro Cruz Garcia's mission of peace. He calls it "Timoteo". That story, however, is for another volume.

Almost two decades have passed since I first walked by the window of an AIDS hospice and felt compelled to help ease the suffering of those dying within. Learning how was not difficult. The methods are, in Dhamodharan's words, "simple and user-friendly". The challenge was in delivering that care. Five years of workshops, another five of clinic operation, and three trips around the world finally distilled a resource as accessible as a phone call or a trip to the fair.

The groups served have expanded far beyond those living with HIV/AIDS, to all who suffer from any cause. When I began, I wanted to deliver hypnosis cassette tapes around the world. Now a common cell phone device that is about the same size can access the online program and provide nearly instant relief. Time, too, is its own force.

In the years since our trip to India, the word "tsunami" itself has undergone a great change. Before the great Asian Tsunami, it was a word somewhat akin to "Godzilla", some unimaginable horror both known and unknown. Since then, our culture has come to define other unimaginable horrors as a "tsunami" of this or that. In 2008, the great financial collapse and resulting recession was expressed as a "tsunami of debt and foreclosures inundating global markets." The "tsunami warning" has become a common report after massive earthquakes have rattled the world in recent years, eventually producing another great wave that savaged parts of Japan. We have come to understand the destructive force of the tsunami and found that to be the only measure by which we can express our own overwhelming circumstances.

In 2008 Lenise and I experienced our own tsunami of loss with the sudden death of our son. Daniel was thirty-two years old and had become my closest male friend as well. He struggled with addiction for several years and as a family we had fought battle after battle, struggling together and wearied from the long ordeal. He had triumphed through treatment and we were planning our future together with him and his son Tobin on the night before I received the unbearable news. He slipped, he fell, and he was gone. The whirlwind of loss sucked the very marrow from the bones of all of us. This hollow, seemingly unendurable sorrow became a surreal altered reality of unimaginable despair.

It was during the long days of that summer that I turned my attention to telling the story of my time in India. On those days that I simply placed my purpose in "turning my face into the hot wind and pressing on," I found strength in the steely resilience of the Tamil village women. It was their determined mission to endure, to provide for their families in the blowing, sandy, tarpaulin tents, and to carry themselves with dignity despite their losses, that encouraged me to move forward each day.

One day while strolling through Srinivasapuram, Dhamu had told me of a tradition held for departed loved ones. Some days after their death, their favorite food is prepared and set out in the open air. If fortunate, the departed will return in spirit in the form of a bird to consume the treat. Lenise and I have watched for and been comforted by such signs from Daniel: a coin appearing on a previously cleared table or floor that is reminiscent of one of his childhood games, a sudden shadow that suggests his profile, or a playlist shuffle that bears significance or stirs a flashback to cherished evenings with our "DJ Danny".

I have tried to explain the feeling of loss that has remained after Daniel's death. It is like a wound that will not fully heal. In time it hurts less, but the sense of loss cannot be quelled, for it will remain all the days of my life. This feeling is akin to the phantom pain of a severed limb, but that missing part is deep within, a part of my heart that has been torn away by the force of irreconcilable separation.

Now some years on, I do not weep quietly within every day. Lenise and I have clung closely together in this journey from rolling rapids to calmer waters and offered comfort to one another. The memory of time together, of laughter, adventures, and "pop and son" challenges saturate my mind and serve as a salve to the wound. Some days, however, when I see a father and son enjoying time together, when I become suddenly mindful of his missing presence during some event we would have enjoyed together, or when I see a lad with his nearly seven-foot tall lanky stature, the old pain returns, like a haunting, carrying me again into the abyss of loss.

It is during these times that I find myself like the bewildered friends in India, like the dispossessed of New Orleans or Moore, like those who have sat in my chair and recounted their struggles through their own great waves of loss. In these times I, like them, seek to feel the comforting touch of a friend, like some great benevolent God reaching out to embrace me and whisper into my soul "tsunami is over; I am here with you, you are safe now."

Acknowledgements

This project could not have occurred without the help of many people. At the top of that list is my beloved wife and partner Lenise Franks Trujillo, my Principle Co-Investigator and Chief Cohort in this life's adventure. Lenise has given direct and moral support to every step of the work, from my initial studies in hypnotherapy, to the development of First Medicines, to working side-by-side during the 2003 European heat wave for three grueling, rewarding weeks at the United Nations in Geneva, to the home station support of the India Tsunami Outreach, etc, etc, etc. Every valued experience in my life since 1983 has been made that much richer because I have had a best friend like Lenise to share it with. Additionally, Lenise helped guide every word in this volume. I will be eternally grateful for her support and help.

Also of immeasurable value was the team that helped to hone the language I wrote down into a more cohesive story. I am especially grateful to my "Three Sisters" whose edited manuscripts guided me from draft to book. They include Debbie Allen's keen pragmatic educator's eyes, Elissa Meininger's knack for storytelling and enthusiastic desire to tell the First Medicines story, and Wilda Spalding's scalpel-like document sculpting that also helped with many other documents, including those presented at the United Nations. It was Wilda that first recognized global value in this work and invited me to share it at her roundtables at the United Nations, where she shepherded me and so many through the UN/NGO process.

Others who reviewed the text and offered valuable feedback include: George Oswalt, N. Dhamodharan, Jim Rudolph, Anne Marie Gillen, Judith Simon Prager & Harry Youtt, Pierre-Etienne Vannier, Terry Weber, & Joe Mattioli, Jamie Lee Nash, Alison Toothman, and Cheryl Cornelsen, my ninth grade English teacher who introduced me to Shakespeare and Poe and has remained a treasured friend and mentor for almost forty years. She was also a principle sponsor in helping to bring this story to print.

I have deep appreciation for the help of Crystal Hawkins in the preparation of the book cover for print, as well as putting the websites timothytrujillo.com and firstmedicines.org in proper order.

It was the team of remarkable individuals that I worked with in India who made my experience there a tale worth sharing. Mitta Wise answered my call for project help in 2002 and worked with diligence to help organize the Hypnosis Health Service Members as a global outreach network. Her heartfelt desire to join me in India helped to transform the team in ways that may not be knowable. Narayanan Dhamodharan's compassion for his people and vision for possibility led our project from a notion to help one community to a mission to serve and transform multiple villages and peoples. This work could not have happened without the assistance of Vijay, Basker, and Dessapan who truly made our individual skills the work of a team. Of course, none of this would have occurred without the confident acceptance of Jim Rudolph to send us to those he so diligently supported and protected. Ryan Geirach's insightful response to two friend's needs initiated the entire enterprise.

Our financial donors truly helped us to realize this dream. I am deeply grateful to Michael Saul, whose generosity fueled possibility. John and Sarah Cooke gave both financial and hospitality support during this project that redefined the boundaries of friendship. Continuing appreciation is sent to the following donors: Marianna Ang, Kathleen Armstrong, Valerie Austin, Nancy Black, Rob Blalack, Elizabeth Burns, Jane Caverly, Raynel Chaves, Kathleen Corcoran, Toni Pace Carstensen, Jethro Carter, Frank Dana, Bud Franks, Renee Gordon, Anne Marie Gillen & Bernie Wire, Delight Hanover, Edgar Iobst & Brian Cheatham, David le'Chastaignier, Helen Macias, Lisa McPherson, George Michela, Anil Mohin, Joseph and Micki Poupolo, Judith Simon Prager, Aneetha Reddy and family, Sandy Reid, Bill Shepard, Pam Shriver, Renee Thiel, Susan Thomas, Bud & Pat Trujillo, Dean Williams, Bobby Young, Arthur Zweig, Michael Weinstein and AIDS Healthcare Foundation, and many others whose contributions were anonymous.

I am thankful to those whose support and counsel helped to guide the development of First Medicines. That list begins with Ormond McGill,

The Dean of American Hypnotists, whose instruction encouraged me to be the very best that I could be as a therapist and whose written and spoken wisdom continues to guide me. My principle hypnosis instructor, Gil Boyne, provided the tools and understanding of trauma recovery that remains the cornerstone of all my work. Charles Farthing, former Chief of Medicine of AIDS Healthcare Foundation, was first known by me as "The Good Doctor" due to the remarkable reports I received from his patients. He became my most ardent supporter and patron of this work in the medical community. His kind heart remains my emblem of quality care. Charles Montagu gave me a sense of the significance of the work and helped me to remember that being a hypnotist is first and foremost a fun-filled adventure. Doug Elliot and I met on a balmy afternoon in Malibu during the California Men's Gathering. I taught him to fold a paper crane and he later guided me in transforming my project operation from an attaché case to an elegant treatment center.

I was also guided by an advisory board whose input helped craft each major step. This board included Barbara Kennedy, Joseph Poupolo, David le'Chastaignier, Cheryl Revkin, Anita Rivas, Michael Sausser, and Buzz Young, who called me in July of 2000 to learn how he could help bring my workshop at APLA to a broader audience. His assistance and persistence is a driving force in my life to this day. Deep thanks also go to Janet Elliot and Community Partners for taking a risk on my fancy ideas.

Finally, it is the staff, volunteers, and network practitioners who transformed my one-man operation into a global endeavor. Thank you Dean Williams, Lisa Hecht, Samantha Grant, Judy Bruissard, Scott Sandman, Joe Poupolo, James Esquer, Jerry Lineback, Mitta Wise, Renee Thiel, Sandy Reid, Jamie Rusche, Brenda Fister, Lucy Irwin, Elizabeth Skala, Fulton & Maki Wright, Pierre Etienne Vannier, Isaac Alfonso & Lucy Penata, and the one hundred thirty-one hypnotherapists in fourteen states and four countries who joined my mission to provide service despite ability to pay to those who suffer serious health challenges.

For every individual working to reduce suffering in every corner of the world, from founder, to clinic or field worker, to office volunteer, thank you for your service. You are the saints of the living world.

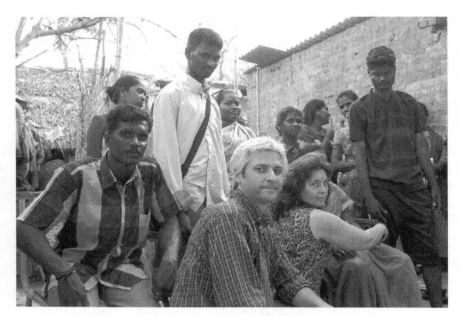

The Team: Vijay, Basker, Timothy, Mitta, Dhamodharan

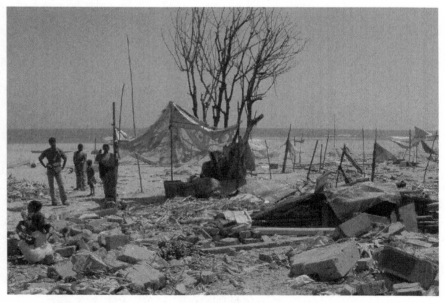

Srinivasapuram Treatment Clinic with Dhamu & Vijay's House Remnants

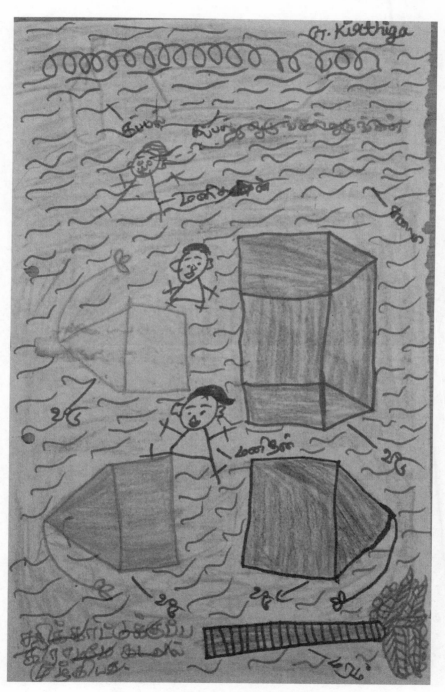

Tsunami artwork from child in Muttkadu

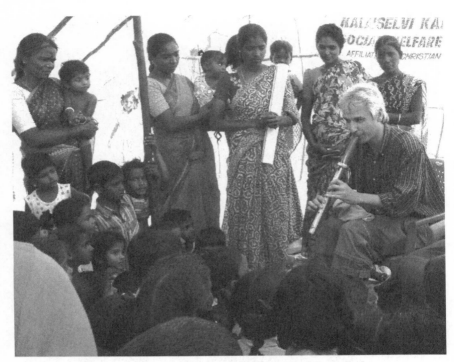

A flute song for students and teachers in Muttukadu

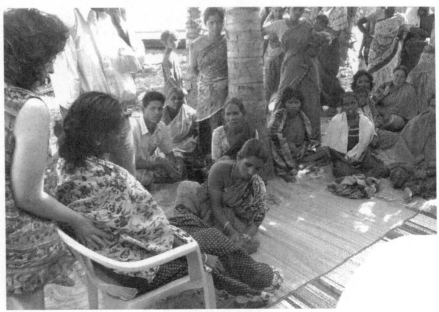

Clinic in Kalapeti

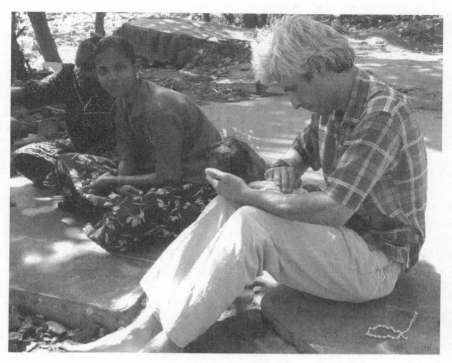

Treating infant with Coué cord in foreground

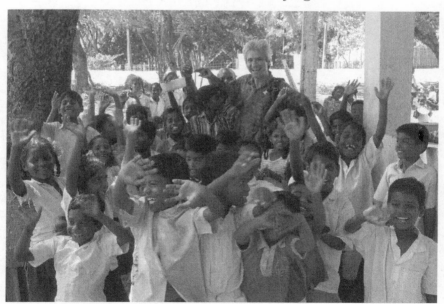

Farewell from the children of Muttukadu

First Medicines
The Five-Minute Miracle

Read slowly aloud to a friend-

Close your eyes and focus on your breathing. Every time you exhale, you naturally relax. Tune into that relaxation and allow yourself to relax more with each exhalation. With each breath you may allow a pleasant color to give you a sense of strength and calm. Allow all the sounds around you, and every thought you have, cause you to relax more. Imagine that you have little faucets attached to your hands and feet. Visualize or imagine those faucets opening wide to allow any tension or discomfort to flow easily out of your body. In your mind visualize, and in your body experience this flow becoming eventually a trickle, and then just a drip. You can also imagine a faucet attached at any location on your body that you feel you would benefit from greater relaxation or comfort now. As you continue to release, just allow every muscle and every nerve to become completely relaxed, comfortable, and at ease. *(pause briefly)*

As you continue to relax, allow a light, airy sensation to flow through you, causing you to feel totally weightless. Allow this sensation to cause you to feel as though you are floating upward, higher and higher, safely tethered, like a helium balloon or kite attached to a long string. As you drift, allow this sensation to cause you to release all cares, concerns, or discomforts. Allow yourself to drift in your mind to a very pleasant place, a place where you feel safe, secure, comfortable, and in complete control. Allow yourself to experience these qualities of safety, security, and comfort in every area of your life. *(pause)*

Now I am going to count from twenty to one. As I do, allow your comfort and relaxation to double with each number. As I reach the number one, allow yourself to settle restfully, right where you are. Allow yourself to remain relaxed and perfectly comfortable from head to toe. 20, 19, 18, now drifting and settling; 17, 16, 15, so relaxed and so at ease; 14, 13, 12, 11, letting calm comfort be yours now; 10, 9, 8…7, 6, 5…4, 3, 2, 1; now let yourself just settle perfectly. *(Allow a few moments of silence)*

Now I am going to count from one to five; as I do, allow yourself to return to full wakefulness. Allow those faucets now to fill you with strength, confidence and well-being and on the number five, allow your eyes to open. One, this calm comfort is always yours. Two, you express it in every area of your life. Three, feel strength moving through you, feel confident and more alert. Four, your eyes now feel as though they have been rinsed in cool spring waters that are refreshing every cell in your body. Five, let your eyelids open, take a deep breath, and feel a peaceful calm throughout your entire body now.

The Coué Method

Tie twenty knots in a string or string twenty beads.
Holding each knot or bead while sitting comfortably,
recite aloud or silently the following:

Every day, in every way, I am better and better.

Hear The Five Minute Miracle
& view the treatment demo video at:

firstmedicines.org/five-minute-miracle

View a full slideshow of photos from India:

timothytrujillo.com/tsunamieffect

Read the original Field Reports at:

firstmedicines.org/field-reports

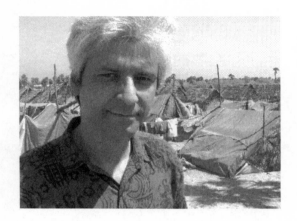

Timothy L. Trujillo is a Mind-Body Healing Specialist. A practitioner of Hypnotherapy, Reiki, Acupuncture, Homeopathy, Reflexology, and Aromatherapy, he is an expert in pain relief, trauma recovery, and immune disorder management. He is one of the world's foremost authorities on the use of hypnosis in the management of HIV/AIDS.

As founder of First Medicines, he has helped to deliver this system of care to HIV/AIDS-impacted populations in Los Angeles since 1996 and has led outreach projects in Guatemala, India, New Orleans, and Cairo, reaching beyond HIV care to address traumatic distress in survivors of tsunami, hurricane, and civil war.

In 2003 he was awarded the Medaille d'Excellence by the International Human Rights Consortium for bringing his "Spirit of Creativity" to the promotion of global health and peace.

Made in the USA
Columbia, SC
19 June 2021